Editors

Dr John Ferguson
Medical Director, Prescription Pricing Authority, Bridge House
152 Pilgrim Street, Newcastle upon Tyne NE1 6SN

Dr Margaret Upsdell
Halton Hospital, Hospital Way, Runcorn WA7 2DA

Contributors

Ms Toni Belfield
Director of Information, Family Planning Association, 2–12 Pentonville Road,
London N1 9FP

Mrs Walli Bounds
Research Coordinator, Research Unit, Margaret Pyke Centre and
Principal Research Fellow, University College London
73 Charlotte Street, London W1P 1LB

Professor Michael Campbell
Professor of Medical Statistics, University of Sheffield, Institute of Primary Care
Northern General Hospital, Sheffield S5 7AU

Ms Ann Furedi
Director of Communications, British Pregnancy Advisory Service
26–7 Bedford Square, London WC1B 3HH

Dr Ailsa Gebbie
Consultant Gynaecologist, Family Planning and Well Woman Services,
18 Dean Terrace, Edinburgh EH4 1NL

Mr Michael Gillmer
Women's Centre, John Radcliffe Hospital, Headley Way, Oxford OX3 9DU

Dr Anna Glasier
Director, Lothian Primary Care NHS Trust,
Family Planning and Well Woman Services, 18 Dean Terrace
Edinburgh EH4 1NL

Professor John Guillebaud
Professor of Family Planning & Reproductive Health, UCL;
Medical Director, Margaret Pyke Centre, 73 Charlotte Street, London W1P 1LB

Professor Philip Hannaford
Director of the Royal College of General Practitioner Centre for Primary Care Research and
Epidemiology, Department of General Practice and Primary Care,
Foresterhill Health Centre, Westburn Road, Aberdeen AB25 2AY

Mr Ali Kubba
Department of Obstetrics & Gynaecology, St Thomas' Hospital
Lambeth Palace Road, London SE1 7EH

Dr Sam Rowlands
Medical Director, The Epidemiology and Pharmacology Information Core (EPIC),
Regeneration House, York Way, London N1 0BB

Dr Gillian Vanhegan
Medical Director, Brook Advisory Centres, 165 Gray's Inn Road, London WC1X 8UD

Key advances in
the effective management

of

Contraception

Edited by

J Ferguson and M Upsdell

Series Organizer
A Miles

Proceedings of a symposium sponsored by Schering Health Care Ltd and held at the Royal Society of Medicine, London, 22nd January 1999

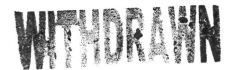

The ROYAL
SOCIETY *of*
MEDICINE
PRESS *Limited*

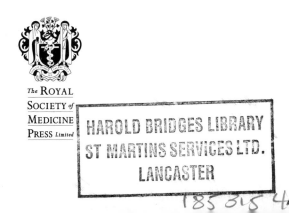

© 1999 Royal Society of Medicine Press Ltd

1 Wimpole Street, London W1M 8AE, UK
207 E. Westminster Road, Lake Forest, IL 60045, USA
http://www.roysocmed.ac.uk

These proceedings are published by the Royal Society of Medicine Press Ltd with financial support from the sponsor. The contributors are responsible for the scientific content and for the views expressed, which are not necessarily those of the editor of the series or of the volume, of the Royal Society of Medicine or of the Royal Society of Medicine Press Ltd. Distribution has been in accordance with the wishes of the sponsor but a copy is available to any fellow of the society at a privileged price.

British Library Cataloguing in Publication Data

A catalogue record for this book is available from the British Library

ISBN 1–85315–422–9

Typeset by Saxon Graphics Ltd, Derby

Printed in Great Britain by Redwood Books, Trowbridge, Wiltshire

Contents

Foreword

The Key Advances symposia held at the Royal Society of Medicine aim to provide a solidly clinical contribution to evidence-based medicine in the UK. Attention is focused on open debate and the contextual interpretation of new medical evidence in a variety of common disease states.

The symposia are intended to facilitate true analysis of the available evidence: practice guidelines, scientific evidence, cost-effectiveness and clinical audit data.

This book presents clinical strategies for the efficient and effective management of contraception. The Guest Editors and Contributors, all distinguished clinicians in their field, are to be commended for their efforts in producing an accessible, highly readable text of immediate relevance to continuing medical education and personal clinical practice.

Professor Andrew Miles
Series Organizer
St Bartholomew's Hospital, London

Preface

Ever since humans became aware of the relationship between intercourse and pregnancy, they have searched for a method (mechanical, medicinal or magical) that could prevent conception or limit the number of children resulting. Planned parenthood is a fundamental human right, and a balance between the population of the world and its natural resources and productivity is necessary for human happiness and prosperity.

The advent of hormonal control of contraception in the closing decades of this millennium fired the imagination of the medical world. It was the first of the 'magic', new methods urgently needed to solve world population problems, and is one of the most effective and acceptable methods to date. So was it the answer to the maiden's prayer? Simple and safe contraception, without complications — the publicity was enormous and expectations were high. However, the oral contraceptive pill has not lived up to all expectations and, as a result of occasional scare stories in the press questioning its medical safety, some women have understandably become cautious in its use.

This book in the Key Advances series provides an up-to-date account of current knowledge in topics relevant to healthcare professionals involved in the provision of modern contraceptive services. The book opens with a historical review, and the initial chapters give an account of the current situation and importance of up-to-date information. Subsequent chapters discuss provision of contraceptive services in general practice and in specialist clinics, along with trends and patterns of prescribing in general practice. There are then updates on hormonal and emergency contraception and non-hormonal methods, and contributions on contraception failure and communication of risks to patients. Finally, there is crystal ball-gazing into the future that the ideal contraceptive will be developed early in the next millennium.

Dr John Ferguson
Medical Director
Prescription Pricing Authority
Newcastle upon Tyne

Historical review

Michael Gillmer, Women's Centre, John Radcliffe Hospital, Oxford

Ignorance has always been the greatest obstacle to effective contraception.

Pre-literate times

Incomplete understanding of the processes leading to pregnancy are typified by the beliefs of the natives of Madagascar who thought a woman, after her first intercourse, would continue to have children whether or not she had further intercourse. This conveniently avoided the need for any form of contraceptive practice. Infanticide was common in some societies, such as that on the Canary Islands, and abortion, although rare, was also attempted.

Herbs have been used for a variety of medical reasons since ancient times — some, by chance, may have had a contraceptive effect. The Cherokee Indians are purported to have used potions made from spotted cowbane roots for contraceptive purposes, although whether or not this or any other potion was effective seems unlikely. Accidental ingestion of grain contaminated with ergot may have produced abortion but it seems unlikely that the cause was recognized.

Douching with a solution of lemon juice and an essence derived from mahogany rusks is reputed to have been used by the women of Guyana and Martinique. This combination was probably highly effective as a spermicide.

Among the Australian aborigines, subincision of the penis, which involved slitting a variable length of the penile urethra, was performed possibly as an initiation rite. In extreme form this caused the semen to dribble over the scrotum during intercourse, thus reducing the likelihood of intravaginal insemination.

Pottery decorations suggest that the Indians of Peru used oral or anal intercourse to prevent unwanted pregnancies — a practice that continues to this day.

The ancient world

Doubt about the nature of pregnancy existed in early civilizations. Thus, while Aristotle believed that women were merely the reservoir for the male essence which contained all that was necessary for reproduction, Hippocrates and Pythagoras were of the view that pregnancy only occurred as a result of union of the male and female.

The *Petri Papyrus* (circa 1850 BC) is believed to contain the earliest medical prescriptions for contraception. One example is the use of a paste-like substance containing crocodile dung as a pessary. A more pleasant alternative included honey and sodium bicarbonate. The *Ebers Papyrus* (circa 1550 BC) included a prescription for pessaries derived from the tips of acacia trees, containing gum arabic. Lactic acid, which is spermicidal, is produced on fermentation. This was combined with honey which acted as an adhesive and barrier.

Hippocrates (?460–377 BC) described a number of techniques for contraception in his book *On the Nature of Women*, including coitus interruptus and the use of fingers to wipe out the vagina. Soranus of Ephesus (98–138 BC), a gynaecologist, obstetrician and paediatrician, described several contraceptive techniques in his book *On Midwifery and the Diseases of Women*. These included ineffective techniques such as breath holding at the time of ejaculation and sitting down with bent knees and sneezing. He, however, also described several ointments to be applied to the cervix before intercourse, including oil, honey or cedar

1

gum, either mixed together or combined with white lead or myrtle oil or alum. While these vaginal applications may have had some contraceptive effect, other techniques including potions of myrrh and pepper or cyrenaic sap and the juice of rue made into a pill with wax swallowed with watered wine, were definitely ineffective. He also mistakenly believed that pregnancy was most likely immediately before or after menstruation. Conversely, he did advocate both douching and coitus interruptus as means of preventing conception.

The Hebrews during captivity in Egypt used a barrier 'sponge' made from Egyptian lint known as 'makk'. This technique was considered acceptable by the rabbis as *man* had been commanded to propagate the human race and *woman* was therefore free to use the 'sponge'. Mixtures of acacia and honey were also used. The Hebrews appear to have been aware of the fertile period, as indicated in Moses's injunction to the children of Israel:

'And if a woman has an issue of her blood she shall be unclean. But if she be cleansed of her issue, then she shall number herself seven days and after that she shall be clean.'

The ancient Chinese methods appear to have used a mixture of sorcery and superstition. These included swallowing 16 tadpoles fried in quicksilver and the advice that women should remain passive during intercourse. They also practised coitus reservatus, ie allowing detumescence to occur immediately before ejaculation.

The Middle Ages

European attitudes during the Middle Ages were profoundly influenced by the Roman Catholic Church, especially in matters relating to sexuality. St Augustine (354–430), in his tract *Marriage and Concupiscence*, condemned contraception even for married couples. St Thomas Aquinas (1225–1274) states in his *Summa Theologica*:

'Insofar as the generation of offspring is impeded, it is a vice against nature which happens in every carnal act from which generation cannot follow. Whenever pleasure is the chief motive for the marriage act, it is a mortal sin; when it is an indirect motive, it is a venial sin, and when it spurns pleasure altogether and is displeasing, it is wholly void of venial sin.'

Islamic religious law during the Middle Ages did not forbid contraception and, as a result, Islamic physicians were free not only to explore scientific means of contraception but also to disseminate their medical knowledge. The scientific giants of this time included Aetios, Al-Rhazi, Avicenna and Ibn al-Jami.

Aetios of Amida (527–565) recommended pessaries using astringents, oil, honey and resins for application to the cervix. He also described methods which were based on pure superstition including amulets, one which contained a child's milk tooth or marble that was to be worn near the anus.

Al-Rhazi (Rhazes), who was born in Persia and died in around 923, described three effective contraceptive techniques in his *Quintessence of Experience*:

'Occasionally it is very important that the semen should not enter the womb as, for instance, when there is a danger to the woman in pregnancy or, if it has entered, that it should come out again. There are several ways of preventing its entrance. The first is that, at the time of ejaculation, the man withdraws from the woman so that the semen does not approach the os uteri. The second way is to prevent ejaculation, a method used by some. A third method is to apply to the os uteri, before intromission, some drug which blocks the uterine aperture or which expels the semen and prevents conception such as pills or pessaries.'

These observations which even today have some practical relevance were combined with advice that was totally irrational, such as the woman performing acrobatic exercises to dislodge the semen or jumping backwards seven times after intercourse.

Avicenna (980–1037) was a famous Islamic physician and philosopher. In his *Canon of Medicine*, he described several methods of contraception which again provide a curious mixture of the scientific and illogical. The latter included avoidance of simultaneous orgasm and violent jumping after intercourse to dislodge the semen and the former, coitus interruptus, insertion of leaves and seed mixed with tar into the vagina and anointing the penis with sweet oil before coitus.

Ibn al-Jami (a Jewish physician at the court of Sultan Saladin between 1171 and 1193) recommended, in *The Book of Right Conduct Regarding the Supervision of the Soul and Body*, smearing the penis with onion juice before intercourse and use of tampons impregnated with peppermint, pennyroyal or leek seeds. He also suggested that eating beans on an empty stomach would be effective.

Reproductive physiology

During the Middle Ages, investigation of reproductive physiology was restricted by Christian teaching which had hitherto explained all nature in deistic terms. Towards the end of the 15th century, however, lay teachers began to gain control over universities and the power of the Church weakened. Despite this, any theory which contradicted Christian dogma was treated with great superstition and this situation undoubtedly stifled scientific development.

This is exemplified by one of the events that followed Antoni van Leeuwenhoek's discovery of the microscope. In 1674, his student, Hamm, observed human spermatozoa for the first time and, in 1677, van Leeuwenhoek gave a detailed description of the appearance of human semen. He stated:

'What I describe here was not obtained by any sinful contrivance on my part, but the observations were made upon the excess with which nature provided me in my conjugal relations.'

He was clearly anxious to avoid the enmity of the Church but was still criticized severely by some.

Rapid progress was made in the 18th and 19th centuries. Although Reinier de Graaf had described the follicle that bears his name in 1672, it was not until 1827 that Carl Ernst von Baer discovered that it contained the mammalian ovum. Further progress occurred in 1841 with the recognition by Rudolph von Koelleker that sperm originated in the testes and in 1843 when Martin Barry observed the union of the sperm and ovum. In 1865, Franz Schweiger-Seidel recognized that sperm contained a nucleus and cytoplasm and, in 1875, Oscar Hertwig observed the sperm enter the ovum. Less than 10 years later, in 1883, Edouard van Beneden discovered that each germ cell had reduced its chromosome complement by one-half.

Population size and the birth control movement

Population control has always been a concern of civilized man. Plato and Aristotle both warned of the dangers of over-population at a time when population size was largely dependent on natural disasters, famine and war.

The first serious consideration of population control in modern times began with the essays of Thomas Malthus (1766–1834), an Englishman who, although ordained in the Church of England, ultimately became Professor of History and Political Economy at the East India Company's College. Malthus' first essay, *On the Principle of Population*, was published in 1798. He highlighted the fact that, while population numbers can increase geometrically, the ability of the earth to provide subsistence for an enlarging population can only occur arithmetically. At this time in England, girls could marry at 12 and boys at 14, prostitution was commonplace, and divorce rare. His solution — later marriage, strict pre-marital chastity and moral restraint — was simple but was unlikely to be effective.

As with the scientific investigation of reproduction, effective advice on contraception was prevented by restraints imposed by the Church. The birth control movement was formed in the early 19th century but its progress was restricted by the moral climate at the time. The first attempts to provide effective contraceptive information were made by Francis Place (1771–1854). He trained as a tailor and ultimately became the owner of an exclusive men's shop in Charing Cross, London. During the day, he served the wealthy and by night, he read, studied and made friends among his intellectual clients. Place was familiar with Malthus' theories but, as a father of 15 children, he knew that moral restraint would not succeed as a means of controlling family and population size. He felt later marriage would increase prostitution, and favoured early marriage as a means of controlling venereal disease. Place was a friend of Jeremy Bentham (1748–1832), an enlightened philosopher and founder of University College London. Bentham introduced Place to the idea of the vaginal sponge and other means of contraception. This inspired Place to write and distribute a handbill entitled *To the Married of Both Sexes* in which he advocated both the 'withdrawal method' and the vaginal sponge. Surprisingly, and despite the fact that his writings were described by some as 'diabolical filth', Place was never arrested.

Place's followers, in particular Richard Carlile, were less fortunate. Carlile was apparently free of any social restraint concerning sexual matters and, in 1826, published *Every Woman's Book: What is Love*. Although considered 'coarse and naïve', this was the first book in the English language that openly discussed the medical aspects of birth control. Carlile was jailed several times on charges of blasphemy and obscenity but, despite this, his book was extremely successful and published in an abridged second edition.

In the late 18th century, attitudes towards contraception remained the same; following the publication by Charles Bradlaugh and Annie Besant of *Fruits of Philosophy*, written by the American physician Dr Charles Knowlton, Bradlaugh and Besant were arrested. The trials took place between 1877 and 1879 and, as a result of Besant's impassioned plea on behalf of the poor, the court found in their favour.

Although the medical profession generally remained hostile to the concept of birth control, in 1887 Dr Albutt, a prominent Edinburgh physician, published the pamphlet *The Wife's Handbook*. Although issues related to pre- and post-natal care were mainly discussed, a section on contraception was also included. This offended Albutt's colleagues and he was subsequently removed from the list of Fellows of the Royal College of Physicians.

Similar attitudes prevailed in the US where, since the founding of the American colonies, matters relating to sex were considered the province of the devil. This puritanical view was also observed in the activities of Anthony Comstock (1844–1915), a dry goods salesman, who in 1879 obtained legislation prohibiting the US postal service from delivering contraceptive information or products, which were categorized as 'obscene materials'. Throughout his life, Comstock maintained a crusade against vice and used entrapment as a means of identifying those involved in the contraceptive trade. He would, for example, write using an assumed woman's name requesting contraceptive material and subsequently arrange for the purveyor to be arrested. Shortly before his death he claimed:

'I have convicted enough to fill a passenger train of sixty coaches containing sixty passengers each, and the sixty first almost full.'

He also claimed to have destroyed 160 tons of obscene material.

The credit for founding the birth control movement in the US belongs to Margaret Sanger (1879–1966), a nurse who devoted her life to providing information about contraception to all women, especially the poor. In 1913, she travelled to Europe to learn about birth control clinics and returned to the US in 1914 with formulae for douche solutions and pessaries. During this time, she met Marie Stopes (1880–1958), a paleobotanist from Manchester, who was subsequently inspired to write the book *Married Love* and to open the first British birth control clinic in London in 1921. No attempt was made to close it down. While the birth control movement was under way in Britain in the 1920s, progress in the US was slow. Stopes' book sold out in two weeks and ran to six editions. In the US, it was banned as obscene.

In 1916 Margaret Sanger opened a birth control clinic in Brooklyn which was closed down 10 days later after an undercover police woman purchased a pessary for $2. Margaret Sanger and her sister were arrested and each sentenced to jail for 30 days. Five years later, she opened a second clinic which prescribed mainly the diaphragm together with spermicidal pessaries. Although Margaret Sanger employed a doctor in this clinic, most of the medical profession ignored her efforts. One exception was Dr Robert Dickinson who, in 1924, read a paper entitled *Contraception: A Medical Review of the Situation* at the 49th Annual Meeting of the American Gynecological Society. He strongly supported Margaret Sanger and defended her from her critics.

In 1936, the Brooklyn clinic ordered a package of Japanese pessaries and Margaret Sanger's lawyer decided to precipitate a test case at law. The package was seized and the case tried before Judge Hand as 'US vs One Package'. He found in favour of the defendants and in his judgement stated that if Congress in 1879 had been aware of the risks of pregnancy and abortion, the Comstock Law would never have been passed.

Between 1935 and 1939, several birth control clinics were opened in the US initially without objection but, in 1939, the state police raided the Waterford Clinic arresting two physicians and a nurse and forcing all other clinics to close. Attempts to reverse the restrictive legislation continued throughout the 1940s and 1950s but were defeated by the attitude of the Senate which was not prepared to risk conflict with the Roman Catholic Church.

In 1961, Estelle Griswald and Professor Lee Buxton (Chairman of the Department of Obstetrics and Gynecology at Yale university Medical School) opened a clinic in New Haven, Connecticut. Shortly afterwards they were arrested and the case was heard by the US Supreme Court who ruled that the Connecticut Birth Control Law was 'unconstitutional'. The Comstock domination finally ended.

Methods of contraception

Barrier methods

The origins of the condom are unknown. A sheath covering the penis is depicted in a tablet from the Egyptian XII dynasty but its purpose is uncertain. It is believed that African women used an okra pod that had been hollowed out as a female condom and Roman women may have used goat's bladder in the same way. The male condom was also known in ancient Rome.

During the Renaissance, sausage skins were used as penile sheaths; Gabrello Fallopia described a linen sheath in 1671.

Condoms were apparently in general use in Europe in the late 17th century and were used by Casanova de Seingalt (1725–1798) both for contraception and to prevent sexually transmitted infections.

Goodyear's invention of the vulcanization of rubber in 1843 improved both the reliability and acceptability of the condom and their use has been widespread for more than a century.

Casanova provided the earliest description of a cervical cap consisting of half a lemon shaped to cover the cervix. It is likely to have been extremely effective as it combined a barrier with a highly spermicidal acid. Much later, in 1838, Frederick Wilde described a rubber cap shaped to cover the cervix and, a few years later, Mesinga designed a 'diaphragm' to cover the cervix which fitted under the pubic symphysis. These methods in their modern versions are still in use but have declined in popularity.

The vaginal sponge was reintroduced in the 1980s as a plastic sponge impregnated with a potent spermicide. However, it is not a popular method due to its poor effectiveness in comparison with other modern contraceptives.

A plastic female condom has also been marketed in recent years but has not been a great success.

Intrauterine contraceptive devices

Camel riders are reputed to have inserted a pebble into the uterus of their camels as the animals apparently become fractious when pregnant — how this was achieved remains uncertain.

Ernst Grafenberg, in 1928, reported on his use of star-shaped devices made out of silkworm gut and later developed a ring made out of 'German silver'. These were not, however, popular as there was a risk of developing pelvic infection, especially during insertion. In the 1930s, Ota in Japan developed a variety of devices including a metal ring and a plastic disc but it was not until the advent of antibiotics that intrauterine devices became widely used.

Since the 1950s, several devices have been conceived with a wide range of shapes, including the Lippes Loop, the Birnberg Bow and the Hall Stone Ring. Following the studies of Zipper in Chile in the 1960s, these inert plastic devices have all been superseded by those containing or made of copper and which continue to be widely used today.

An active device, the Progestasert, was marketed in the 1970s but was unpopular due to the need of its annual replacement. More recently, the Levonova, which releases the progestogen levonorgestrel, has been introduced. This can remain in situ for five years and is rapidly becoming more popular: it is more effective than previous devices and is unique in reducing, rather than increasing, menstrual blood loss.

Combined oral contraceptive pill

The earliest demonstration that fertility could be influenced by hormonal manipulation is attributed to Ludwig Haberlandt of Innsbruck who, in 1921, performed ovarian transplants between pregnant and non-pregnant animals of the same species, rendering them infertile. Around the same time, Otfried Fellner, working in Vienna, reported infertility in rabbits following injection of a lipid extract of the ovary which he called 'Feminin'. Much later, in 1937, Makepeace and co-workers in the US reported inhibition of ovulation in rabbits following progesterone ingestion, while in 1940, Sturgis and Albright, also in the US, reported inhibition of ovulation in women with dysmenorrhoea treated with oestradiol injections.

Shortly before this in 1938, Hans Inhoffen, a German chemist in Berlin, had produced a potent synthetic oestrogen, ethinyloestradiol, and the progestogen, ethisterone, by the addition of an acetylene group at the 17-carbon position of the naturally occurring hormones oestradiol and testosterone, respectively.

Subsequently in 1942 an enigmatic chemist Russell Marker, who was Professor at the State College in Pennsylvania, managed to synthesize progesterone from the root of the wild Mexican yam. The following year he joined two Hungarian émigrés, Dr Emeric Somlo and Dr Frederico Lehmann, who owned a small pharmaceutical company in Mexico City and founded Syntex (a name derived from the words *synthesis* and *Mexico*) in 1944. Five years later, Carl Djerassi joined the company and, in 1951, used the same plant source as Marker to remove the 19-methyl group from Inhoffen's ethisterone, producing the highly potent and orally active progestogen, norethisterone.

The previous year, Gregory Goodman Pincus, the 'father of the pill', had been introduced by Margaret Sanger to the wealthy heiress Mrs Katherine McCormick. Both women had impressed on Pincus the need for new contraceptive techniques, especially for the women of the third world, and it is reputed that the idea of an oral treatment was considered at this time. In 1952, Searle filed a patent for the progestogen, norethynodrel.

The first clinical study of these progestogens was initiated in December 1954. Preliminary results demonstrating inhibition of ovulation were presented by Pincus at the 5th International Planned Parenthood Conference held in Tokyo in October 1955. Paradoxically Japan remains one of the few countries in the world that has not yet licensed the combined oral contraceptive pill. A field trial using norethynodrel began in Puerto Rico early in the following year. It is of interest that one of the major reasons for selecting Puerto Rico for these studies, rather than the US, was the strong opposition to birth control that still existed in North America at this time.

The original intention had been to study the pure progestogen norethynodrel but this was subsequently found to contain the oestrogenic contaminant, mestranol, in amounts ranging from 0.08 to 0.23%. When the oestrogen was removed, cycle control became a problem and pregnancies occurred. It was therefore reintroduced in a dose equal to the average of the contaminants (0.15%), thus producing, purely by chance, the first combined oral contraceptive, Enovid, containing 0.15 mg mestranol and 10 mg norethynodrel.

Enovid was licensed by the US Federal Drugs Agency (FDA) for the control of menstrual disorders in 1957 and as a combined oral contraceptive in 1960. It is of interest to note that in the context of the preceding millennia, the evolution of the 'pill' from laboratory to the market place took less than a decade.

In Britain, trials of the pill started in Birmingham in 1960 and a lower dose preparation, Conovid, was licensed in early 1961. It was not, however, until 1962 that Djerassi's progestogen norethisterone was marketed. Ironically, it is the only early progestogen still used in oral contraceptive pills and it is now accepted that norethynodrel is in fact converted in vivo to norethisterone by the weak acid in the stomach.

Conclusion

A clearer understanding of the physiological processes of reproduction is fundamental. Ignorance among individuals is the main problem in achieving population control even today.

Further reading

1. Gillmer MDG. The pill: an historical overview. In: Hannaford PC, Webb AMC, eds. *Evidence-guided prescribing of the pill*. Carnforth: The Parthenon Publishing Group Ltd, Carnforth, 1996: 15–27.
2. Robertson WH. *An illustrated history of contraception*. Carnforth: The Parthenon Publishing Group Ltd, 1990.
3. Speert H. *Obstetric and gynecologic milestones*. Carnforth: The Parthenon Publishing Group Ltd, 1996.

Presenting the problem

Philip Hannaford, Department of General Practice and Primary Care, Foresterhill Health Centre, Aberdeen

During the past 40 years, there has been an astounding increase in the use of contraception around the world, from about 10% of all couples of reproductive age in the early 1960s to more than 50% by the 1990s.[1] This reproductive revolution has resulted partly from the introduction and improvement of a number of contraceptive methods. Combined oral contraceptives and plastic intrauterine devices became available in the 1960s, modern tubal ligation, vasectomy and copper intrauterine devices in the 1970s, and longer-acting subdermal implants in the 1980s. During the 1990s, a progesterone-releasing intrauterine device and the frameless intrauterine implant (Gynefix) have been introduced. There have even been technological advances in the humble barrier method of contraception: female condoms have become available, as have plastic versions of the male condom.

Other factors have contributed to the increased uptake of contraception. Users, particularly women, have appreciated that control of their fertility allows them to improve their standard of living. Governments have become aware that sustainable global development is only possible if human population is restricted. The emergence of the human immunodeficiency virus (HIV)/acquired immune deficiency syndrome (AIDS) pandemic has highlighted the additional need for protection against sexually transmitted infections.

In addition to the expansion of the range of contraceptive choices, there have been improvements in the safety and side-effect profile of individual methods. This is partly a result of technological developments. For instance, the hormonal content of combined oral contraceptives has decreased over the years. Improved safety has also resulted from increased knowledge of risks and benefits of the different contraceptive methods, in particular from greater understanding of which users may be prone to an adverse event. For example, it is known that most (if not all) of the cardiovascular risks associated with combined oral contraception occur in users who: smoke, have high blood pressure, or have not had their blood pressure checked before using the pill.[2] This type of information enables service providers to carefully select and monitor those wishing to use a particular method of contraception.

Factors influencing choice of method

In spite of all these major advances, the perfect reversible contraceptive (100% efficacious in preventing pregnancy, immune to user and provider failure, no clinically significant side-effects, no adverse effects on health, cheap to produce and provide, aesthetically acceptable) remains an Utopian dream. The imperfections of currently available methods are reflected in recent research that suggests women's choice of contraception often continues to be a matter of selecting the 'least worst' option.

In December 1995, an independent market research company interviewed, on behalf of the Contraceptive Education Service run by the Family Planning Association and the Health Education Authority, a random sample of 744 women aged 16–49 years living in Britain.[3] Three-quarters of the women interviewed had used more than one reversible method of contraception; 13% had used four or more different reversible methods. More than one-half of those women who changed their most recent method had done so following their experience of a side-effect or health problem, or because of worry about perceived health risks (Table 1). Other reported problems included difficulty in using the previous method correctly, receipt of new information about effectiveness, side-effects or health risks of the method, and concerns about the effectiveness of the method in protecting against pregnancy. When these women were asked about possible reasons for choosing a contraceptive method, absence of health problems, contraceptive efficacy, fewer side-effects and ease of use were deemed to be the most important.

Table 1 Reasons for women changing their method of contraception[3]

Reason	% women
Experience of a side-effect/health problem	56
Worry about perceived health risks	53
Difficulty in using previous method correctly	49
New information about effectiveness, side-effects or health risks	48
Concern about effectiveness in preventing pregnancy	46

It is important to note that this survey was conducted just after the last 'pill scare' relating to possible differences in venous thromboembolic risk between users of different combined pill formulations. This may have affected the responses of women who had been using the contraceptive pill. There were also differences in perceived importance of reasons for changing contraceptives between users of the different methods. Nonetheless, it is probably true that negative factors — concerns about side-effects, health risks, and possible ineffectiveness in preventing pregnancy — still strongly influence contraceptive choice and use.

Ambivalent attitudes to contraception are suggested by high discontinuation rates and frequent switching both within and between methods. Fears about side-effects and health risks can result in women choosing methods that are less effective in preventing pregnancy. These concerns can also contribute to incorrect and inconsistent use of the selected method, thereby increasing the chances of unintentional pregnancy. Twenty-seven per cent of former pill users and 36% of former condom users in the UK survey reported becoming unintentionally pregnant while using the respective method.[3]

Role of the media

Many contraceptive users do not have sufficient knowledge of both contraceptive methods and services. Much information comes from the media and, unfortunately as far as contraception is concerned, the news is usually (although not inevitably) bad. There are a number of reasons why this should be the case. First, contraception is inextricably associated with sexuality, which is still a difficult subject to discuss openly in some sections of society. Exaggerated or false concerns about safety are sometimes used to try and force a greater restriction on the availability of contraception, presumably in the hope that this will reduce sexual activity. Second, most contraceptive users are young and healthy and are using a product to prevent an unintentional pregnancy rather than to treat a disease. Many will be using their chosen contraceptive for many years. As a consequence, contraceptives need to have exemplary safety profiles, possibly better than those associated with medical treatments to treat disease. The huge number of users means that small increases in risk of common disorders result in many individuals being affected. In addition, any major adverse events that do occur, however rarely, are liable to be viewed as particularly poignant tragedies. Third, there are still no agreed, clear ways of presenting scientific knowledge about safety that is understandable without being misleading. For example, results from epidemiological studies are often presented in terms of relative risk alone without consideration of absolute (attributable) risk which provides more meaningful information about the clinical significance of any finding. In addition, it is sometimes forgotten that much epidemiological research is concerned with the average risk across all users, information that may not represent (indeed may mislead) the particular risk of an individual using a contraceptive.[4] An important reminder of this point is the example of concentration of arterial risk in combined contraceptive pill users who smoke, have high blood pressure or who have not had their blood pressure checked. Finally, there may be an inevitable bias in the reporting of the safety of all preventive services so that reports of adverse events predominate. This is because those who benefit from the measure (such as women who do not develop ovarian or endometrial cancer because of their use of combined oral contraception) do not know that they were at risk in the first place. Conversely, those who experience an adverse event are aware that the event has occurred. Bad news sells newspapers and attracts viewers and listeners, whereas good news usually does not.

Given these powerful influences, it is perhaps unrealistic to hope that there will be no more media scares in the future. Clinicians can, however, counter some of their effects by ensuring that users have as much accurate information as they need when choosing and using contraceptives. Access to the latest information at the time of a media scare can also reduce anxiety and re-establish confidence in the contraceptive method. Unfortunately, current information about the risks and benefits of contraception often contains mixed messages. For example, a contraceptive is sometimes said to be very safe, although the potential user is simultaneously subjected to a number of clinical tests. Such contradictions lead to users, and the media, asking why these tests must be carried out if the particular method of contraception is so safe.

Variation in clinical practice

Clinical practice is also inconsistent. In a survey of contraceptive providers, 95% of 123 attendees at the Third Congress of the European Society of Contraception in 1994 stated that they checked the blood pressure of all or most women before prescribing combined oral contraceptives.[5] There was, however, less agreement with regard to other practices: two-thirds stated they weighed all or most potential pill users beforehand, and around one-third examined women's breasts or pelvic organs.

The general agreement about blood pressure probably reflects strong, consistent evidence that combined oral contraceptives can raise the blood pressure of some women, and that blood pressure is directly related to risk of stroke or heart disease.[2] The disagreement about the value of other procedures possibly stems from tacit recognition by clinicians that some aspects of their clinical practice are not based on good evidence. It may also represent different levels of knowledge among the clinicians.

In their defence, it is important to acknowledge that all clinicians have the increasingly difficult task of acquiring, maintaining and incorporating comprehensive up-to-date information into their work. Clinicians providing contraceptive services are no exception. Indeed, it could be argued that they have a special need for accurate up-to-date information. The large number of contraceptive users means that any procedures deemed obligatory before a method can be prescribed affects many women. Unnecessary medicalization of the consultation process can have major impacts on the accessibility and acceptability of contraceptives.[6] Other opportunity costs can result from unnecessary interventions, eg reduced opportunities to discuss choice of method, correct usage, safer sex and other aspects of reproductive well being. Inappropriate screening can convert a carefree user of preventive services into a worried patient. Avoidance of a method because of unsubstantiated health concerns may deny the potential user important benefits. For instance, women denied combined oral contraception lose the opportunity to benefit from a substantial, long-term protection against ovarian and endometrial cancer.

In the absence of time (and possibly skills) to identify, read, digest and interpret all the scientific evidence for themselves, many clinicians rely on expert opinion. Such opinion also shapes some of the other influences on clinical practice: undergraduate and postgraduate teaching, recommendations from professional and recognized experts, fear of litigation, previous experience, method of remuneration, commercial pressures from industry, cultural attitudes towards curative and preventive medicine, and the personalities and prejudices of all parties concerned. Unfortunately, expert opinion can be surprisingly subjective. Review articles, for instance, may only discuss published data and the thoroughness of the literature search may be variable, diminishing the validity of the conclusion reached.[7]

Expert opinion can also be inconsistent. For example, the authoritative *Handbook of Contraceptive Practice* includes the statement that 'vaginal examinations, repeated at regular intervals, form the basis for good preventive care',[8] whereas in the opinion of another expert group the available evidence strongly suggests that this procedure should not be performed in asymptomatic women.[9] In another example, multiple sclerosis is said to be a relative contraindication to use of a combined oral contraceptive,[8] a special precaution,[10] a condition requiring careful observation during usage,[11] or is not mentioned at all.[12]

To address these and other deficiencies, researchers around the world are trying systematically to review and scientifically summarize all the available relevant information. While very welcome, this work will always only address one dimension of clinical practice. Caring medical practice will remain a blend of both art and science. To this end, expert opinion and the views of consensus groups will continue to be needed. What will be increasingly unacceptable, however, will be proclamations and recommendations without the backing of scientific evidence (or at least without an acknowledgement when such information is not available).

Conclusion

It is probably unrealistic to believe that the negative factors influencing contraceptive choice and use can be entirely overcome. Choice of contraception is highly dependent on the confidence users have with both the method selected and the service provider. Such confidence can be increased by obtaining information. There is a need for a better understanding of how accurate, up-to-date, understandable and comprehensive information can be effectively disseminated to, and used by, both users and providers of contraceptive services. This information challenge remains one of the major barriers preventing the optimal use of contraceptive services throughout the world.

References

1. Anonymous. Family planning — public policy, private needs. In: Marshall A, ed. *The state of world population 1994 — choices and responsibilities*. New York: UNFPA, 1994: 21–30.
2. WHO Scientific Group on Cardiovascular Disease and Steroid Hormone Contraception. *Cardiovascular disease and steroid hormone contraception*. Report of a Scientific Group. WHO Technical Report Series 877. Geneva: World Health Organization, 1998.
3. Walsh J. Contraceptive choices: supporting effective use of methods. In: Ravindran TKS, Berer M, Cottingham J, eds. *Beyond acceptability: users' perspectives on contraception*. Geneva: World Health Organization, 1997: 89–96.
4. Hannaford PC, Owen-Smith V. Using epidemiological data to guide clinical practice: review of studies on cardiovascular disease and use of combined oral contraceptives. *BMJ* 1998; **316**: 984–7.
5. Owen-Smith V, Hannaford P, Webb A. What do family planning providers do before prescribing combined oral contraceptives? *Br J Famil Plann* 1996; **22**: 103–4.
6. Shelton JD, Angle MA, Jacobstein RA. Medical barriers to access to family planning. *Lancet* 1992; **340**: 1334–5.
7. Mulrow CD. The medical review article: state of the science. *Ann Intern Med* 1987; **106**: 485–8.
8. Department of Health. *Handbook of contraceptive practice*. London: Department of Health, 1990.
9. Hannaford PC, Webb AMC on behalf of participants at an international workshop. Evidence-guided prescribing of combined oral contraceptives: consensus statement. *Contraception* 1996; **54**: 125–9.
10. Duncan C (ed). *Monthly index of medical specialties (MIMS)*. London: Haymarket Medical Ltd, August 1996: 260–1.
11. Anonymous. *ABPI data sheet compendium 1995–1996*. London: Datapharm Publications Ltd, 1995: 1145, 1159, 1161, 1164, 1603, 1605, 1606, 1608, 1613, 1615, 1622, 1629, 2000, 2004, 2020, 2022.
12. Anonymous. *British national formulary*. London: British Medical Association and Royal Pharmaceutical Society of Great Britain, 1997.

Sources of information

Ailsa Gebbie, Family Planning and Well Woman Services, Edinburgh

Both providers and consumers of family planning services in the UK have a requirement for up-to-date information on contraception. This paper addresses the sources of contraceptive information relevant to these two groups.

For providers of contraceptive services

The providers of contraceptive information are primarily general practitioners (GPs), practice nurses, family planning clinic staff and other healthcare professionals working in obstetric, gynaecological and genitourinary medicine departments. Traditionally, healthcare professionals obtain information on new developments from original and review articles published in medical journals.

Published work

Journals

In the UK, the only dedicated journal on contraception is the *British Journal of Family Planning*, the journal of the Faculty of Family Planning and Reproductive Healthcare, which has a circulation of around 9,500 in the UK. A small number of other publications cover contraception in the sexual health context and are funded mainly through grants from pharmaceutical companies. Internationally, there is a small selection of dedicated contraceptive journals mainly originating in North America, such as *Contraception* and *Family Planning Perspectives* — these only have a relatively small circulation in the UK.

Occasionally, articles on contraception of major importance appear in mainstream general journals such as *British Medical Journal*, *Lancet*, *New England Journal of Medicine* and *Journal of the American Medical Association*. In 1996, the *British Medical Journal* had only two original articles, three editorial articles, nine letters and five news items on contraception. The *Lancet* had two original papers, nine letters and 17 news items on contraception. For comparison, there were 24 articles on alcohol abuse and more than 100 articles on human immunodeficiency virus (HIV) and acquired immune deficiency syndrome (AIDS) in the *British Medical Journal* in 1996.

With the major advances in research over the past two decades, it has become increasingly difficult for healthcare professionals to assimilate new information. Over two million health research papers are published in more than 20,000 biomedical journals annually. An average consultant would need to read 19 articles per day, 365 days of the year, in order to keep up-to-date — most British consultants on average spend less than one hour per week reading. With this 'information nightmare', an accessible, straightforward and useful summary of the best evidence is required. Research findings need to be translated into simple, easy-to-read, high quality reviews that are based on the best available evidence.

Books

Books remain a valuable source of reference for healthcare professionals. Books about contraception vary from pocket-sized handbooks to large, authoritative texts. GPs frequently cite the value of the *Handbook of Family Planning and Reproductive Health Care* as a quick reference tool.[1] However, in a rapidly developing area, with the inevitable delays incurred during the preparation and publication of textbooks, books fail to keep pace with important new developments.

Media

Generally, the media is a less important source of information for health professionals than for contraceptive users. However, major items of information about contraception may appear in the popular press before reaching medical or nursing staff by any other route. The 'pill scare' in October 1995 is an example. Details of new drug therapies, including new methods of contraception, may also appear in newspapers before being disseminated widely in medical journals.

Cochrane Collaboration

In 1979, Archie Cochrane, a British epidemiologist and clinical trialist, argued that, given limited resources, only forms of care that research had clearly shown to be beneficial should be offered by the National Health Service (NHS). The randomized controlled trial was the form of research most likely to yield reliable estimates of the effects of care. In response to this, the Cochrane Collaboration, an international network of individuals and institutions, is attempting to address this need for reliable, summary information.

In 1992, the Cochrane Centre was funded as part of the research and development programme developed to support the NHS. The following year, the initiative was launched internationally as the Cochrane Collaboration with further Centres in Australia, Canada, Italy, Scandinavia, the Netherlands, France and the US.

The aim of the Cochrane Collaboration is to prepare, maintain and disseminate systematic reviews of randomized controlled trials on the effects of healthcare. Against a background of putting family planning on a robust scientific foundation, the Fertility Regulation Group of the Cochrane Collaboration has been formed. This group addresses:

- processes by which people regulate their fertility, family size and spacing of births
- efficacy and safety of fertility-regulating measures
- delivery of services
- how people obtain and use information
- how people make and implement choices about fertility regulation
- issues relating to policy development.

In addition to using electronic search databases such as Medline, the Cochrane Collaboration has established a controlled trial register by rigorously hand searching all previous issues of journals. Reviews, along with the database of all randomized controlled trials in family planning, are expected to be available soon in electronic CD format in the Cochrane Library — the CD is issued quarterly and presented in a standardized, graphic, easily comprehensible format. The reviews will also be published in traditional medical journals. It will be made known where no reliable information is available on a particular intervention.

Faculty of Family Planning and Reproductive Healthcare

The Faculty of Family Planning and Reproductive Healthcare was established in 1993 with the aims of:

- enhancing clinical knowledge about family planning
- providing education and training for doctors in the field
- promoting high standards of professional practice.

It is the only professional body for doctors working in the field of family planning in the UK. The Faculty's Clinical Effectiveness Committee maintains a scientific database of advice for members and develops evidence-based clinical guidelines, eg on emergency contraception.[2] The Faculty supports the National Coordinating Unit for Clinical Audit in Family Planning, which is based at the University of Hull. *Audit Unit* newsletters and recommendations for clinical practice are regularly disseminated to members.

In the context of reaccreditation for the Faculty of Family Planning, courses and meetings that address new developments are held regularly.

Family Planning Association

Following integration of free family planning services into the NHS in 1974, the Family Planning Association's current role lies in the field of public information and education, as well as training and providing support for professionals. The Contraceptive Education Service (CES) is a national contraception information service for the UK, run by the Family Planning Association in partnership with the various Health Education Authorities.

Electronic sources

Several Internet sites relating to contraception have been established in the UK for healthcare professionals. These include an e-mail discussion forum and web site for evidence-based practice in family planning, and a collection of family planning resources with links and access to Medline. Links can also be made to other web sites concerned with evidence-based family planning such as the Human Reproduction Programme of the World Health Organization (WHO) and Family Health International. The e-mail addresses concerned are HYPERLINK http://www.nthames-health.tpmde.ac.uk/ebfp/ and HYPERLINK http://www.nthames-health.tpmde.ac.uk/Family_PlanNet.[3]

A CD ROM teaching package recently developed for GPs (by the Royal College of General Practitioners and Scottish Council for Postgraduate Medical and Dental Education) includes a programme on family planning. This Phased Evaluation Project (PEP) in Family Planning, comprising multiple choice questions and a patient management problem, is designed to discover strengths and weaknesses in the field and provide a stimulus to continuing medical education. By completing the programme through self-assessment, GPs gain points for their postgraduate education allowance (PGEA).

For consumers of contraceptive services

Healthcare professionals

Almost all GPs provide contraceptive advice. Most family planning in the UK currently takes place in the primary care setting. All general practices are now required to produce leaflets describing the contraceptive services they offer. A widespread network of NHS family planning clinics also operates to provide contraceptive services and specialist advice on contraception.

Leaflets and books

An excellent range of patient information leaflets on contraception is available in the UK in a variety of languages. The Family Planning Association provides the most comprehensive range of leaflets, but many pharmaceutical companies also produce detailed information sheets. It is widely acknowledged that patients often have a poor recall of verbal instructions given to them regarding the combined oral contraceptive pill; written data can reinforce this information. A study from Bristol showed that leaflets on the combined pill and emergency contraception significantly increased the level of knowledge on the '12-hour rule' and 'seven-day rule' for the pill, and the duration of effectiveness for emergency contraception.[4] Questioning of the patient by the doctor, in addition to providing a summary leaflet, is time-consuming but women taking the combined pill gain most knowledge and information in this way.[5] Books on contraception for the lay public are widely available, generally competitively priced and accurately written.

Interactive computer programmes

Touchscreen patient education systems are an innovative way of educating patients on medical topics, including contraception. They are an information delivery system which is objective, non-threatening and allows the user complete control over how fast the information is delivered. Graphical images and voice-overs can be incorporated in addition to text. Standardization of the information given to patients is guaranteed. Such systems have already been installed in some GP surgeries and have been used successfully in sexual health clinics for young people. Initial costs of setting up these systems can, however, be high.

Friends and family

Word of mouth from friends and family is a long established source of information on contraception. Many myths and taboos about various contraceptive methods have been perpetuated in this way and have affected uptake and use of particular methods, such as Depo-Provera and intrauterine devices.

Media

Television, radio, newspapers and magazines are all extremely important sources of information on contraception. Women's magazines particularly focus on aspects of women's health including contraception. Much of what appears is inaccurate and sensationalized by journalists. Recently, advertisements by lawyers coordinating litigation against several methods of contraception have been appearing regularly in the national press and encouraging the public to sue for 'damages'.

The Internet

The Internet has grown rapidly over the past five to 10 years and its use extends globally. A vast free market of information is potentially available to Internet users in many areas, including healthcare. Poor quality health information is found on the Internet, but very little is known about epidemiology in medical information and it is hard to identify which information processes lead to unfavourable health outcomes. The WHO has convened a group to recommend that nations act together to control cross-border advertising, promotion and sale of medical products through the Internet. The possibility of somehow labelling health information is being examined in order to set information standards and use technology to help the public sift good information sources from bad.[6]

A large number of web sites relating to contraception can be readily accessed using various search engines. These sites are predominately North American and include pharmaceutical companies, contraception and abortion clinics, university departments, journals, books, chat lines and interactive web sites. Electronic information is unique in that it can be infinitely duplicated at minimal cost and very cheaply distributed. It is simply not known to what extent the Internet is being used as a source of information in contraception but it seems highly likely that it will play an increasing role in the future.

Helplines

Telephone helplines are popular with consumers as they provide a rapidly accessible and anonymous source of information. The CES has a telephone helpline service in addition to a wide range of publications and a library/information centre. It handles over 100,000 enquiries each year by a telephone, postal and personal enquiry service. The NHS helpline provides free and confidential information on all aspects of healthcare in the UK, including details of services available for contraception.

Conclusion

Sources of information on contraception for both providers and consumers are numerous and extremely diverse. Traditional medical literature is at risk of becoming quickly out-dated and, eventually, of being superseded by rapidly accessible electronic sources of information. Although the media plays a very prominent role as an information source, it is often inaccurate.

References

1. Loudon N, Glasier A, Gebbie A, eds. *Handbook of family planning and reproductive health care*. London: Churchill Livingstone, 1995.

2. Kubba A, Wilkinson C. *Recommendations for clinical practice: Emergency contraception*. London: Faculty of Family Planning and Reproductive Health Care, 1998.

3. O'Brien P. The Cochrane Collaboration: preparing, maintaining, and disseminating systematic review in fertility regulation. [Editorial]. *Br J Famil Plann* 1997; **23**: 37–8.

4. Smith LF, Whitfield MJ. Women's knowledge of taking oral contraceptive pills correctly and of emergency contraception: effect of providing information leaflets in general practice. *Br J Gen Pract* 1995; **45**: 409–14.

5. Little P, Griffin S, Kelly J *et al*. Effect of educational leaflets and questions on knowledge of contraception in women taking the combined contraceptive pill: randomised controlled trial. *BMJ* 1998; **316**: 1948–52.

6. Coiera E. Information epidemics, economics and immunity on the internet. [Editorial]. *BMJ* 1998; **317**: 1468–9.

Provision of services: general practice

Sam Rowlands, The Epidemiology and Pharmacology Information Core (EPIC), London

Despite technological advances in contraception, at least one-third of pregnancies in the UK are unintended. This paper will focus on improving the quality standards of contraceptive care in general practice, in order to keep unintended pregnancies in the community at the lowest possible level.

Primary healthcare team

General practice no longer solely refers to general practitioners (GPs). The primary health-care team (PHCT) provides the service: the core team involved with contraception includes practice nurses, receptionists, the practice manager, health visitor and midwife; the wider team includes the school nurse, pharmacist, social worker and counsellor. The team model should be moving from the autocratic GP leader to a more democratic, shared leadership.[1]

The service depends on a well-functioning team, which is likely to have the following qualities:

- a common goal or vision for the team
- respect and understanding of members' varying skills and knowledge, including the uniqueness of their roles
- support and development for individual roles
- ability to listen to team members and to patients' views and concerns
- acceptance and management of conflict.

Teams have to pass through the forming, storming and performing stages of any group[2] and an outside facilitator can be very helpful during this development process.

Relevant statistics

Women tend to favour GPs as their primary source of contraceptive advice (Figure 1).[3] In England, approximately 75% of contraceptive advice is given in the setting of general practice (Table 1);[4] this proportion has risen from 46% over the past 15 years, probably due to clinic cutbacks and the increased emphasis given to contraception by the PHCT. Obviously, the accuracy of these figures is questionable as there is considerable overlap of use of general practice and family planning clinic services in any one year. The proportion seeking contraceptive advice from their general practice is much lower for very young women: a study in Oxford in 1991–2 revealed only 39% of users aged under 16 to have consulted a GP.[5]

A survey of women aged 20–49 years in a single rural practice showed 30% choosing methods of contraception that are not medically dependent (Table 2);[6] it can be expected that some of those choosing an over-the-counter method would seek the advice of pharmacists.

There is a serious lack of information about the male partner's role in the use of contraception.

Premises and equipment

Curtains drawn around couches to provide privacy when undressing should be the norm.[7] Use of the Family Planning Association leaflets available without cost from Health Promotion Units is best practice as they have been vetted by experts, written by professional writers and consumer tested. Use of leaflets has been shown to improve knowledge of pill rules in a randomized controlled trial.[8] Locally produced leaflets may well not meet these criteria.

19

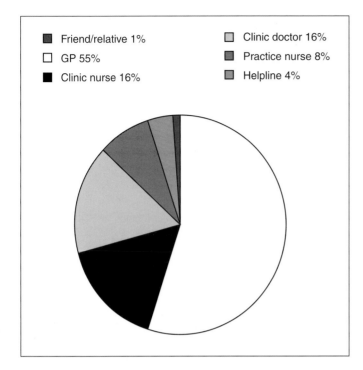

- Friend/relative 1%
- GP 55%
- Clinic nurse 16%
- Clinic doctor 16%
- Practice nurse 8%
- Helpline 4%

Figure 1: Source of contraceptive advice preferred by women.
Redrawn and reproduced with permission[3]

Sterilization of instruments must meet EU and British standards. Same-day pregnancy testing should be available.

The practice nurse

Practice nurses are often underused and undervalued; their potential for giving family planning advice is enormous. In some practices, there seems to be a lack of awareness that the role of the practice nurse has moved on from the treatment room nurse who is the GP's hand-maiden. Greater assertiveness is now needed on the part of the nurses to point out what they can contribute, and less resistance from GPs to expansion of their role and of joint working practices.

Reasons for patients choosing to consult the practice nurse about family planning and related matters include:

- the nurse is female
- the nurse is known to a parent because she has carried out the children's immunizations etc
- the patient may 'try out' the nurse with a problem, asking if it is something she should 'see the doctor about'
- some patients prefer to discuss their problems with a nurse, feeling that the nurse is less threatening than the doctor
- other PHCT members may suggest to a patient that the nurse is the appropriate person to see.

Practice nurses often work in a more flexible way with their appointment systems and are usually seen as more accessible than GPs. Telephone advice is an important part of their work and can save patients a lot of time. Many women prefer to have their barrier method fittings and checks with a nurse. However, it is essential that nurses do not work outside their sphere of competence. Nurse services often need to be more actively promoted. A recent publication by the Contraceptive Education Service is a highly recommended resource for practice nurses.[9]

Staff training and qualifications

A survey of GPs in Wessex found that those GPs who held the Joint Committee on Contraception (JCC) certificate offered a wider range of contraceptive services than those who did not (Table 3).

Table 1 Family planning activity, England: 1994–5[4]

Family planning clinics: number of women seen	1,092,200
General practice: number of women registered for contraceptive services	3,521,700
Total	**4,613,900**

The JCC certificate was superseded by the Diploma of the Faculty of Family Planning (DFFP) with the formation of the Faculty of Family Planning and Reproductive Health Care in 1993. Since then, almost 11,000 diplomas have been issued, mostly to doctors working in general practice.

Nurse training in what is termed family planning and reproductive sexual healthcare (FP&RSH) is undergoing change. The English National Board (ENB) 901 is defunct and appropriate qualifications are now:

- foundation programme: four weeks ENB9903 — this is very long for an introductory course
- practice of FP&RSH: 16 weeks ENB8103 (or R71 based on Lancaster Health Authority's own version) — this course is also long. Nurses who complete it are in many respects better qualified than a GP with the DFFP.

A group practice may wish to have one nurse with the ENB8103 or equivalent.

Receptionists need specific training on how to judge which requests are urgent (particularly important for timely access to emergency contraception) and telephone skills.

A comprehensive service

Despite the fact that 80–90% of women attending general practice for contraception are prescribed oral contraceptives,[10] ideally all prescription methods of contraception should be available. These include: hormonal emergency contraception, implants, injectables, intrauterine devices, intrauterine systems, spermicides, and diaphragms and caps.

Practices should strive for a system that provides male condoms too; many practices have been able to organize this, for instance by using arrangements with their health authority. If a method has not historically been provided by a practice, a good exercise is for the PHCT to produce a 'spider' diagram with reasons for non-provision, and solutions as to how any resistance can be overcome and the method introduced or arrangements made for easy referral to a nearby service.[1]

There should be familiarity in the PHCT with other methods of contraception and how to access them locally, such as: Persona from pharmacists, female condoms from trust clinics or pharmacists, vasectomy usually from GP colleagues or local trust or private sector clinics, and female sterilization from hospitals.

It is important that local services are integrated so that individuals requesting and suitable for a particular method are not denied access to free contraception.

Complementary to other local services

Good relationships are needed between general practice and community trust clinics. Some areas of the UK benefit from Brook clinics. Directors of clinic services can provide support in the form of telephone advice, training and updating and joint publicity for local services. Other healthy alliances are needed with genitourinary medicine, Accident and Emergency, school nurses and pharmacists.

Table 2 Current source of contraceptive supplies in one rural practice in 1992 (n=825)[6]

Source	% supplies
Own GP	59
Over-the-counter	26
Family planning clinic	11
Mail order	2
Other	2

Table 3 GP holders (n=268) and non-holders (n=130) of JCC certificates offering contraceptive services[7]

	% Holders	% Non-holders
Injectables	94	76
Checking IUDs	95	59
Fitting IUDs	82	39
Fitting diaphragms	74	31
Fitting caps	35	15

IUD – intrauterine devices

In the new primary care group (PCG) environment, liaison with other practices in the PCG will of course be mandatory. Although local policies will be determined for all practices, there will still be competition between practices for patients and so new working arrangements will evolve.

Emergency contraception on Sundays?

The ability to provide this service was recently raised by the World Health Organization.[11] It was shown that both PC4® and the progestogen-only method (Postinor) have greater efficacy when given under 24 hours from intercourse. Not all studies show this but, nevertheless, some service managers are going to want to offer quicker access to emergency contraception. Women exposed on Saturdays need to be offered treatment on the Sunday, rather than asking them to come in on Monday morning. With new, out-of-hours arrangements (either deputizing or cooperatives), more GPs are likely to find it acceptable to offer this kind of service, particularly as duty doctors are on the move or in an emergency centre rather than at home.

Young people

Few teenagers view general practice as their preferred source of contraception (23% of females and 9% of males in a study carried out in 30 schools).[12] According to the teenagers, features that would make general practice services easier to use are: shorter waiting times for appointments, friendlier receptionists, more sympathetic doctors and longer consultations. Young people favour less formal services, are very concerned about confidentiality and have strong feelings about not being judged or patronized. My personal view is that to create a suitable environment in a surgery is a nigh impossible feat. Saturday morning sessions have met with limited success in some surgeries.[7] Ideally, young person's centres should be situated away from premises run according to a medical model.

Even if such an environment cannot be emulated, it is important to be receptive to the needs of those young people who do come to general practice. The flexibility to be able to consult with one or more of the young person's friends, reassurance given on a first visit that confidentiality will be honoured, and explanations given for asking personal details may seem small points to a health professional but make a great difference to helping young people feel comfortable and able to return to the service.

A dedicated clinic or not?

Whatever the decision on this, most family planning advice is woven into general surgeries. Often it takes up part of a consultation that has several components; it may be on the patient's agenda or raised opportunistically by the health professional.[13] The average number of National Health Service GP consultations is 6 per person per year[14] — practice nurses have their own consultations for which there are no data; like all aspects of health covered in consultations by the PHCT, much activity is spread over many separate consultations.

A practice may appoint a doctor or nurse to take the lead on contraception. It may be decided to run a special clinic to which internal referrals can be made. There is, perhaps, a danger in thinking that the presence of such a clinic will automatically raise the overall standard of contraceptive care. Protocols need to be developed and owned by the whole PHCT and applied to general surgeries if standards are to be raised.

Publicity and promotion

An entry in the practice leaflet[15] and posters on notice boards are fundamental. New services or changes in services can be publicized in a practice newsletter. Coordination of arrangements with other local services is more likely to meet people's needs. Joint advertising may be useful. General Medical Council guidance on advertising is clear — as long as information is factual and verifiable, and one's own services are not compared with those of other practices or clinics, there is freedom to advertise widely.[16]

Use of outcome indicators

Quality of contraceptive services can be measured by patient interviews, eg looking at knowledge or satisfaction after consultations. However, true outcome involves counting pregnancies. The PCG is an ideally sized population to study — large enough to give statistical validity and small enough to be a locality to apply relevant policies to. Outcome indicators are not too hard to calculate if the practice is computerized and data entry is of a good standard. Four outcome indicators have been developed by public health specialists to show the effectiveness of the service.

- Total period legal abortion rate (TPLAR). This represents the average number of terminations of pregnancy (TOPs) that would occur per woman if women experienced the PCG's age-specific abortion rates of the calendar year in question throughout their childbearing age span of 15–44 years. The TPLAR was 0.4 for England and Wales in 1986;[17] ie, the likelihood of a woman having a TOP during her reproductive life was 40%.
- Total period legal abortion rate as a percentage of the crude potential fertility rate. The total period fertility rate (TPFR) is the average number of live births that would occur per woman in the PCG if women experienced the PCG's current age-specific fertility rates throughout their childbearing age span. The TPFR runs at about 1.8 in England and Wales, which is equivalent to family size if adoptions are ignored.

   The TPLAR can be calculated as a percentage of the crude potential fertility rate, as follows:
   TPLAR (0.4) + TPFR (1.8) = crude potential fertility rate (2.2)
   (TPLAR (0.4)/crude potential fertility rate (2.2)) x 100 = 18%.

- *Proportion of TOPs performed after 12 weeks' gestation.* This is 11% for England and Wales.
- *Conception rate for those aged under 16 years.* This is 8/1,000 for England and Wales. The Health of the Nation target was to have been 4.8/1,000 by 2000.

The aim is to keep all four indicators as low as possible; this is more difficult in areas with higher deprivation indices.

Looking to the future

There are various ways of limiting the number of unintended pregnancies in the community. It is predicted that these strategies can be improved and further enhanced as listed below:

- Nurses are likely to have a higher profile in the future: the Crown Committee is expected to issue guidance on prescribing powers for suitably trained nurses in due course.
- Pharmacists will be giving wider advice, not just about Persona.
- PC4 and progestogen-only emergency contraception will be available from nurses and pharmacists according to protocols agreed locally by the medical profession and ultimately will be reclassified from prescription only medicines to pharmacy only.
- Medical abortions using mifepristone will extend into the community — the Secretary of State for Health will approve certain family planning clinic premises for this purpose.

References

1. Anonymous. *RCGP Handbook of sexual health in primary care.* London: The Royal College of General Practitioners, 1998.

2. Johnson DW, Wolcott D. *Joining together: group theory and group skills*. London: Allyn and Bacon, 1994.

3. Walsh J, Lythgoe H, Peckham S. *Contraceptive choices – supporting effective use of methods*. London: Family Planning Association, 1996.

4. Anonymous. *Health and personal social services statistics for England*. London: The Stationery Office, 1998.

5. Allaby MA. Contraceptive services for teenagers: do we need family planning clinics? *BMJ* 1995; **310**: 1641–3.

6. Rowlands S. Contraceptive use in a rural general practice. *J R Soc Med* 1998; **91**: :297–300.

7. Rowlands S. *Managing family planning in general practice*. Oxford: Radcliffe Medical Press, 1997.

8. Little P, Griffin S, Kelly J *et al*. Effect of educational leaflets and questions on knowledge of contraception in women taking the combined contraceptive pill: randomised controlled trial. *BMJ* 1998; **316**: 1948–52.

9. White S. *Supporting effective contraceptive use*. London: Health Education Authority, 1998.

10. Walsh J. Changes in the provision of family planning services. *Trends Urol Gynaecol Sex Health* 1998; **October**: 31–4.

11. Task Force on Postovulatory Methods of Fertility Regulation. Randomized controlled trial of levonorgestrel versus the Yuzpe regimen of combined oral contraceptives for emergency contraception. *Lancet* 1998; **352**: 428–33.

12. Donovan C, Mellanby AR, Jacobson LD *et al*. Teenagers' views on the general practice consultation and provision of contraception. *Br J Gen Pract* 1997; **47**: 715–8.

13. Rowlands S. Analysis of the family planning consultation. In: Montford H, Skrine R, eds. *Contraceptive care: meeting individual needs*. London: Chapman and Hall, 1993: 204–19.

14. Thomas M, Walker A, Wilmot A, Bennett N. General health and use of health services. In: *Living in Britain – results from the 1996 General Household Survey*. London: The Stationery Office, 1998.

15. Marshall MN, Pereira Gray DJ, Pearson V *et al*. Promotion of family planning services in practice leaflets. *BMJ* 1994; **309**: 927–8.

16. Anonymous. *Good medical practice*. London: General Medical Council, 1998.

17. Clarke M. Fertility and legal abortion in England and Wales: performance indicators for family planning services. *BMJ* 1988; **297**: 832–3.

Provision of services: specialist services

Gillian Vanhegan, Brook Advisory Centres, London

Patients should have a choice of places to go to obtain advice on sexual health and contraception. The options include: the patient's own general practitioner (GP), registration with another GP for contraceptive services only, community family planning clinics, and specialist young peoples' services, such as Brook Advisory Centres.

Choice in service provision

Over recent years, an increasing number of GPs have become interested in providing this service for their patients — others do not want to or maybe only one partner in the practice will run a special surgery for family planning. It is an advantage to the patient to see a doctor who knows her background, personal and family medical histories. The disadvantage is that some patients are not comfortable with discussing personal, sexual issues with their family doctor. One such example is a young girl who recently attended the centre and said 'I cannot talk to my doctor about contraception — he has known me since the day I was born as he delivered me!'. A more serious case was that of the 24-year-old patient who attended Brook recently. Her family doctor had been prescribing the pill for her since she was 16 and, at each check visit, she had been unable to tell him that she had never been able to consummate her relationships as she had profound vaginismus.

Registering with another GP for family planning is rare in my experience.

The advantage of attending the community clinic is that the patient will see a doctor who is interested in contraception and sexual health and who has a postgraduate qualification in the subject, usually the Diploma of the Faculty of Family Planning (DFFP) or, in the case of the lead clinician, the Membership of the Faculty of Family Planning (MFFP). Doctors will also have Letters of Competence (LOC) in intrauterine techniques, implants and postgraduate education. The patient is offered the whole contraceptive menu and counselling services (Table 1), as far as local funding allows. Health authority funding of family planning services is very variable, eg in London, it is possible to obtain an implant or intrauterine system in one clinic, but not in a nearby one funded by the adjacent health authority. The advantage to doctors is that a substantial amount of teaching is carried out in community clinics.

Over the past few years, funding bodies have failed to appreciate the value of the community family planning services and severe cuts in them have been enforced. Community funding has been directed towards services for the under 25s, while older patients are directed more towards GP services.

A service for the young

Brook Advisory Centres is the only national organization that provides a network of services throughout the UK providing advice on sexual health and contraception to the under 25s. Every year at Brook, 170,000 consultations with young people take place; in the past year, 10,000 new male clients used the service. The majority of clients are under 20, 12% are under 16 and an increasing number are younger teenagers. It is vital to have a specialist service for young people, as around one in three under 16s have had sex and less than one-half will have used contraception on that first occasion.[1]

Sadly, many young people feel that they have been pressurized into having sex by their partner, peer group and the media, and regret it. Young people's centres have not been established to distribute condoms and encourage people to have sex, as critics believe. Such

Table 1   Range of services offered by community family planning clinics

• Barrier methods: male and female	• Termination of pregnancy counselling and referral
• Hormonal methods: oral, injection and implant	• Well women and well men sessions
• Emergency contraception: hormonal and intrauterine	• Contraceptive problem sessions
• Intrauterine contraception: intrauterine devices, systems and implants	• Psychosexual consultations
• Natural family planning	• Sexual health advice
• Sterilization counselling: male and female	• Youth sessions
• Preconception advice	

centres aim to help the young person to analyse the situation and decide what is right for them as an individual, so they make the right choice. First-time sex is also associated with alcohol or drugs use which lower inhibitions. This should be discussed with the young person. One example is the pregnant 14-year-old client who recently attended the centre; she knew she had had sex with someone at her friend's party, but she had no idea who he might be as there had been drugs and drink circulating. This client represents the high number of unintended teenage pregnancies seen in the UK.[2] There is also an increasing incidence of sexually transmitted infections, especially Chlamydia. Young clients need to be advised on these issues.

It is important to deliver a young person's service in a way that is acceptable to young people themselves. In the past few years, three useful studies have been conducted to determine how young people wish the service to be delivered. The studies were carried out at the University of Bristol,[3] Southampton University[4] and Brook.[5] The studies revealed that young people wanted services to be: free, easily accessible, delivered by welcoming, nonjudgemental staff, and under an umbrella of complete and absolute confidentiality.

The Brook study is called *Someone with a smile would be your best bet*, as this was a telling phrase used by a young man in one of the focus groups when referring to going to a centre for advice. It is so important for reception staff to welcome the young client and give them their full attention. The reception area needs a secluded place where the young person can be taken for triage, by a nurse or a specially trained receptionist, as a young person does not want to talk about their need for emergency contraception or a pregnancy test in the waiting area with other clients listening.

The following points should be considered when setting up a young persons' service:

- publicity
- situation and accessibility
- timing of sessions
- appointments or walk-ins
- atmosphere
- staff
- consultation
- confidentiality.

Publicity

A specialist young person's service needs to be publicized so that the young person knows where to attend and what the service offers. If posters and publicity materials are to be meaningful to young clients, it is important to involve young people in the design process. The teenagers in local schools, colleges and youth groups benefit in taking part in this as they will also learn about the service, which might be useful to them at a later date. Posters should be displayed in all local schools, colleges, youth centres, clubs and other places of interest to young people; fliers are useful for distribution in sixth-form goodybags, at freshers' fairs and pop festivals. Young people will also look in local telephone directories and on the Internet for local services.

Situation and accessibility

A specialist service is most acceptable to the user group if it is situated near the main shopping area or high street but not directly on it, so that the client feels he or she can visit with some degree of discretion. It must not be positioned in a 'no go' area for any particular ethnic group or in a homophobic area which would deter gay youngsters from using the service. The building should be made accessible to wheelchair users and the staff trained to help disadvantaged clients, such as deaf people. In order to make it accessible to all young people, the service should also be taken out of the building to hostels for the homeless, sixth-form colleges and rural areas.

Session times

A service for young people is most valuable to them at times when they are free to attend, eg lunch breaks, after school or college at 3–6.30pm, and all day on Saturdays, but not starting too early. A Sunday service is important for the provision of emergency contraception, but it is difficult to obtain funding for this.

Appointments or walk-ins

The needs of young people are very immediate: they often come in a crisis situation requiring emergency contraception or a pregnancy test, so an appointments system does not suit them. They would prefer to walk in and use the service when they need it, even if it sometimes means that they have to wait for a while. The term 'walk-in' is preferred to 'drop-in', as young people say that dropping in is something that their granny does when she comes round for a chat and a cup of tea with their mum.

Atmosphere

The welcoming attitude of the staff should also be expressed in the user-friendly style of the waiting area, which should have posters and reading materials appropriate for young people. They appreciate comfortable chairs, a soft drinks machine and, if funds allow, a television set.

Staff

While the doctors and nurses sitting in their consulting rooms might be approachable and nonjudgemental, it is important to remember that it is the reception staff whom the clients meet first. In the view of young people, staff must be friendly without being nosy and they must not make it difficult for the youngster to see the medical staff. They must have a good telephone manner and be able to encourage the young person to attend the service.

Consultation

The client is often shy or embarrassed and it may take time for the medical staff to ascertain their needs. They will often come to the centre in groups or accompanying a friend, so that they can see what the medical staff are like before they present their own problem. The consultation can take quite a long time and the doctor or nurse has to prioritize the infor-mation to be given in response to the client's needs. For example, if a young girl attends for emergency contraception, as well as discussing emergency contraception, assessing her risk and explaining how to use it, it will be necessary to find out why she needs it and if she might need ongoing contraception. Maybe she is not in a relationship and is distressed by what occurred and she might be at risk of sexually transmitted infections. There is a vast amount of information to give a young person and the staff must be careful not to overload them. All advice should be supported with leaflets in simple language that can be easily understood if the young person is able to read.

Confidentiality

This is the most important issue for young people. They are often concerned about who will

Table 2 Gillick competence: guidelines for assessing young people[6]

Doctors should particularly consider the following isues when consulted by people under 16 for contraceptive services:

- whether or not the patient has the maturity to understand the potential risks and benefits of the treatment and the advice given
- the value of parental support must be discussed. Doctors must encourage young people to inform parents of the consultation and explore the reasons if the patient is unwilling to do so. It is important for persons under 16 seeking contraceptive advice to be aware that, although the doctor is legally obliged to discuss the value of parental support, the doctor will respect their confidentiality
- the doctor should take into account whether or not the patient is likely to have sexual intercourse without contraception
- the doctor should assess whether or not the patient's physical or mental health or both are likely to suffer if the patient does not receive contraceptive advice or supplies
- the doctor must consider whether or not the patient's best interests would require the provision of contraceptive advice or methods or both without parental consent

have access to their notes, or whether or not test results will be sent to their home address and possibly opened by somebody other than themselves. All doctors seeing patients under 16 years of age should be aware of the guidelines for assessing young people attending the centre without parental consent, ie the assessment of Gillick competence. It is important to remember that the duty of confidentiality owed to a person under 16 is as great as that to any other person.[6] Posters stating confidentiality should be displayed in the waiting area to ensure the young client is aware that a confidential service is being provided. Leaflets should also be given to clients. The policy of confidentiality can be reiterated at the beginning of the consultation.

Conclusion

Several factors should be taken into consideration when designing a specialist service for young people. A service for young people does not stop at the door of the centre but continues in advocacy work for young people, representing their needs whether it be to members of parliament, fellow health professionals or to service funding bodies.

References

1. Wellings KJ. *Sexual behaviour in Britain; the national survey of sexual attitudes and lifestyle*. Harmondsworth: Penguin, 1994.
2. *ONS Birth Statistics [England and Wales] Series FM1. Department of Health, Statistical Bulletin 1996/7.* London: HMSO, 1997.
3. West J *et al*. Young people and clinics: providing for sexual health in Avon. A report to Avon health. Department of Sociology: University of Bristol, 1995.
4. Ingham R *et al*. Promoting young people's sexual health services. Health education authority, Brook & University of Southampton, 1996.
5. A qualitative research report on young people's needs and expectations of sex advice services. *Someone with a smile would be your best bet*. London: Brook Publications, 1999.
6. Guidance issued jointly by the BMA, GMSC, HEA, Brook Advisory Centres, FPA and RCGP. *Confidentiality and people under sixteen*. London: BMA Publications, 1994.

Trends and patterns of prescribing in general practice

John Ferguson, Prescription Pricing Authority, Newcastle upon Tyne

Every day, millions of women reach out for a pill pack and swallow a tiny tablet that changes the course of their lives. Many women have done this at some stage in the past, and millions more will do so in the future. More than three million women in the UK currently use the combined oral contraceptive pill. It is the first-choice method for one-half of the women using contraception between the ages of 20 and 24 years. More than 90% of sexually active women under the age of 30 have taken the combined oral contraceptive pill at some stage in their life.

Choice of contraception is important in family planning. In the UK, 70% of women using contraception receive this from their general practitioner (GP), while the remainder use community family planning clinics and specialist clinics for young people. There is no doubt that these sources of family planning advice are complementary. The Prescription Pricing Authority data are derived from general practice prescribing. This paper will, therefore, focus on the trends and patterns of contraceptive prescribing in general practice only.

Development of the pill

As early as 1921, Haberlandt indicated that extracts from the ovaries of pregnant animals might be used as oral contraceptives. In 1937, Kurzrok noted that ovulation was inhibited during treatment for dysmenorrhoea with ovarian oestrone and he suggested that this hormone might be of value in fertility control. It was only with the advent of steroid chemistry that potent progestogens became available and an oral contraceptive pill became possible. In 1943, Russell Marker produced pure progesterone from diosgenin which was extracted from Dioscorea, the wild Mexican yam. In 1951, using the same raw material, George Rosencrantz and Carl Djerassi produced the first orally active progestogen, norethisterone. Initially, these hormones were used for the treatment of various gynaecological disorders.

Pinkus, Chang and Rock found that these new hormones were very effective contraceptives and produced no immediate or obvious harmful effects. They first worked with animals and then used a small group of human volunteers in Boston. In 1956, trials with a larger number of women began in Puerto Rico. These trials were successful until chemists produced highly purified hormones. Immediately things began to go wrong, as the impurity they had removed was ethinyloestradiol. It was this chance finding that demonstrated that some oestrogen is necessary for maximum effectiveness and cycle control.

In 1960, the US Federal Drugs Agency licensed the first combined oral contraceptive pill, Enovid. This contained much higher doses of hormones than are now routinely used. It was introduced in Britain two years later and, for some time, its use appeared to be associated with only minor side-effects which were accepted by most women in return for its high effectiveness.

Since its introduction, the composition of the pill has changed significantly. The total dose of steroid has been reduced, ethinyloestradiol has largely replaced mestranol, some progestogens have been abandoned and newer ones introduced. Further attempts to reduce total steroid content led to the introduction of phased preparations, whose use is limited by their effect on cycle control.

Pill scares

Over the years, there have been occasional scares about the safety of the oral contraceptive pill, which have usually resulted in a temporary reduction in use.

The Committee on Safety of Medicines (CSM) was set up under the Chairmanship of Sir Derek Dunlop following the thalidomide tragedy. Working for the CSM, Bill Inman pioneered the 'Yellow Card' scheme for the reporting of adverse drug reactions. This scheme proved its worth by detecting the problem of thromboembolism with the high-dose oral contraceptive pill.[1] I vividly remember, as a young doctor working as a locum in a rural practice, hearing the warning on the radio and wondering how to deal with the patients and their problems on that particular day. On that same day, I was consulted by three women who firmly expressed their belief that they wished to continue using the pill for its beneficial effects, regardless of the side-effects that had been announced. Immediately, the dosage of oestrogen was reduced to 50 μg or less and pills were reformulated to comply with the advice of the CSM.

Third-generation combined oral contraceptives

On 18th October 1995, the CSM issued a warning on third-generation combined oral contraceptives and thromboembolism.[2] The CSM had become aware of three as yet unpublished epidemiological studies on the safety of oral contraceptives in relation to thromboembolism.[3-5] These studies all indicated that combined oral contraceptives containing desogestrel and gestodene were likely to be associated with around a twofold increase in the risk of thromboembolism compared with those containing other progestogens. There was insufficient evidence to determine whether or not norgestimate was also associated with an increased risk of thromboembolism.

The way in which the CSM presented the new data concealed the relative safety of third-generation pills, as measured by event-free women, from 99.993% for other pills to 99.985% for third-generation pills. The CSM received a lot of adverse comment from the profession over the content of the warning and the way in which it was transmitted. Analysis of the now published evidence certainly supported the stand which the CSM took over desogestrol and gestodene. There has been some speculation that at least part of the problem may have been caused by women with risk factors such as increased age, smoking or obesity having been specifically prescribed third-generation pills.

There has been much speculation and anecdotal evidence in the medical press about the effects of the 1995 warning from the CSM. Some doctors appear to have experienced a major increase in their workload, with women wanting to consult, while for others the problem has been much less. No matter how warnings of this sort are announced, some women are likely to panic and some will stop taking oral contraceptive measures immediately without seeking medical advice. There is then the risk of unwanted pregnancies and a rise in the abortion rate has been announced by the British Pregnancy Advisory Service. Improved methods for communicating these warnings to the profession must be found for the future so they have the information in a timely fashion before the public is alerted.

In April 1999, the restrictions placed on third-generation pills in 1995 were lifted by the CSM, following further review of the available evidence.

Impact on oral contraception use and cost

Since the CSM's warning in October 1995, the Prescribing Pricing Authority has been monitoring the use of oral contraceptives.[6] The proportion of third-generation oral contraceptives containing desogestrol and gestodene, which previously accounted for 55% of the usage and 70% of costs, fell dramatically to about 12% and 23%, respectively (Figures 1 and 2). The main change was towards second-generation pills, which increased from 30% to 62% by usage and 16% to 44% by costs. Though their total usage was maintained in the short-term, there has since been a reduction of 10% in oral contraceptive usage.

Second-generation pills are significantly cheaper than third-generation pills. There has, therefore, been a marked reduction in the costs of oral contraceptives. Recently, the costs of some oral contraceptives have been revised upwards.

The average prescription for an oral contraceptive was for 4.5 months, suggesting roughly equal numbers of prescriptions for three and six months. Following the CSM's warning in 1995, the average prescription length dropped to 3.9 months, which suggests that prescribers were trying new products for a shorter period. It is now returning to its previous level.

Recent trends in use

The national usage chart shows a quarterly use of nine million months' treatment per quarter. Combination products account for nearly 90% of this total, with those based on ethinyloestradiol 30 µg per dose accounting for nearly two-thirds of this total.

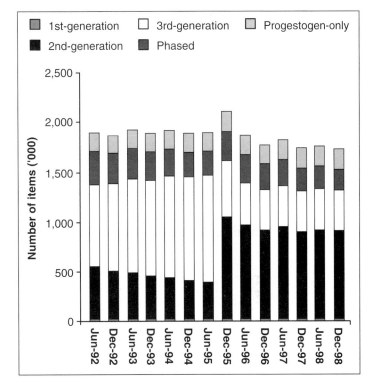

Figure 1: Trends in oral contraceptive prescribing in the UK: 1992–8.

Redrawn and reproduced with permission[6]

First-generation pills now have insignificant national usage and cost. Second-generation pills have shown a slow but steady decline in usage and costs over the past three years, but there has been a marked change in this pattern since the CSM advice of 1995. Third-generation pills had steadily increased in usage and, in overall cost and, for many doctors and patients, were clearly the pill of first choice — their use has shown a marked reduction of some 50% since the CSM advice.

Across the 100 health authorities in England, there is a 1.9-fold variation in the use of the combined oral contraceptive pill, which demonstrates that it is a widely accepted standard treatment.

The use of low-strength pills has halved since 1995 and currently are used by only 120,000 women. Across the health authorities there is a fivefold variation in their use with Cambridge, Kingston and Richmond, and Oxford near the top and Sefton, North Staffordshire, and Barking and Havering near the bottom.

Phasic preparations are slowly declining in usage, possibly due to the better cycle control offered by the third-generation pills. They are currently used by some 373,000 women and there is a 2.4-fold variation between health authorities, with South Humberside and Bedfordshire near the top and West Sussex and Barnet near the lower end.

Progesterone-only pills continue to be fairly constantly used by 280,000 women. There is a 3.4-fold variation in usage between health authorities with Portsmouth, Oxford, Hampshire and Berkshire near the top and Wigan, Walsall, St Helens and Sefton nearer the lower end.

Depot contraception has been available for a long time in the form of Depo-Provera but initially its usage was restricted to short-term. Norplant was introduced in 1993 and had short-term popularity, peaking at the end of 1994 and then declining steadily. This may be due in part to the problems with insertion, use and removal of the rods — as a result, manufacture has now ceased. In 1995, Mirena, an intrauterine device impregnated with

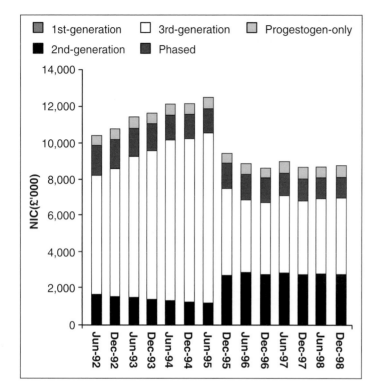

Legend:
- 1st-generation
- 2nd-generation
- 3rd-generation
- Phased
- Progestogen-only

Figure 2:
Trends in oral
contraceptive
spending in the
UK: 1992–8.
Redrawn and
reproduced with
permission[6]

levonorgestrel was introduced and its usage is steadily increasing. Overall, there is a 4.7-fold variation in depot contraception between health authorities with Wiltshire, Tees and Leeds near the top and East Surrey, Barnet , Kensington, Chelsea and Westminster near the lower end. Mirena shows a 17-fold variation in usage, with Shropshire, Somerset and West Surrey near the top and Liverpool, St Helens and Sandwell near the lower end. There is an eightfold variation between health authorities in intrauterine device usage, with East London, Redbridge and Waltham, Brent and Harrow, and Bexley near the top and Norfolk, Wirral, Sefton and Liverpool near the lower end.

PC4® usage shows a slow but steady increase over the years with no peak following the CSM warning, and instead peaking in the quarter ending September 1996. Currently, 150,000 packs are dispensed quarterly and there is a 2.6-fold variation between health authorities with those in inner-London near the top and Sunderland, Barnsley and Walsall near the lower end.

Conclusion

Prescribing trends are changing. The Deputy Chief Medical Officer in the UK has recently announced new guidance for the Medicines Commission that third-generation oral contraceptives can be used first-line, provided the patient is aware of potential risks, following consultation with her doctor. Ironically, the New Zealand government recently announced that, as a result of the safety profile, third-generation oral contraceptives should not be used in the first instance. Nevertheless, the Prescription Pricing Authority will continue to monitor GP prescribing with renewed interest.

References

1.   The Committee on Safety of Medicines. Adverse Reactions Series No 9 – Oral Contraceptives 13 December 1969: London.

2.   The Committee on Safety of Medicines letter 'Oral Contraceptives and Thromboembolism' of 18 October 1995: London.

3.   WHO Collaborative Study of Cardiovascular Disease and Steroid Hormone Contraception. Effect of different progestagens in low oestrogen oral contraceptives on venous thromboembolic disease. *Lancet* 1995; **346**: 1582–8.

4.   Jick H, Jick SS, Gurewich V *et al*. Risk of idiopathic cardiovascular death and non-fatal venous thromboembolism in women using oral contraceptives with differing progestagen components. *Lancet* 1995; **346**: 1589–93.

5. Spitzer WO, Lewis MA, Heinemann LA *et al*. Third-generation oral contraceptives and risk of venous throm-boembolic disorders: an international case-control study. Transnational Research Group on Oral Contraceptives and the Health of Young Women. *BMJ* 1996; **312**: 83–8.

6. Prescribing analysis and cost (PACT) data. Prescription Pricing Authority: Newcastle upon Tyne, 1998.

Why does contraception fail?

Ann Furedi, British Pregnancy Advisory Service, London

Despite careful use, all contraceptive methods have a failure rate. The 1982 Oxford/Family Planning Association (FPA) study (which is still cited as a key reference for efficacy) found that common methods of contraception had a significant failure rate, even when used by participants: over 25 years of age, in long-term relationships, of above average socio-economic status, and sufficiently motivated to return to be interviewed by a research assistant every six months (Table 1).[1]

A more recent study based on data from the US National Survey of Family may present a more accurate picture of contraceptive failure (Table 2).[2] This study reflects a more typical pattern of contraception use by the sexually active population in general.

Method failure versus user failure

The difference between 'method failure' and 'user failure' is frequently discussed, and is explained in client information literature. It is sometimes difficult for those involved in reproductive healthcare services to accept the extent of 'user failure' and to understand why individuals, many of whom manage to lead otherwise ordered lives, fail to use contraceptives effectively.

Studies suggest that contraceptive failure is responsible for a significant proportion of unintended pregnancies. Fleissig's study revealed that 69% of women who had become unintentionally pregnant claimed to have been using a method of contraception at the time they conceived.[3] A study of 769 women requesting abortion on the National Health Service (NHS) revealed 68% of participants claimed to have conceived as a result of a failure of contraceptive method.[4]

Condom failure is frequently cited as a cause of unwanted pregnancy — studies have shown around 48% of abortion seekers claiming such failure.[5,6] Failure of oral contraception is also frequently blamed. One study revealed that, of 1,020 women referred for abortions, one-fifth claimed to have been using the pill — one of the methods regarded as being most effective.[7]

These studies may overestimate the use of contraception at the time of conception, as women seeking abortion may be reluctant to admit that they had unprotected sex in case their request is viewed less sympathetically. However, anecdotal accounts from staff at British Pregnancy Advisory Service clinics suggest that some women are reluctant to admit to contraceptive failure believing the doctor might think them foolish or incompetent. Embarrassment about becoming pregnant in these circumstances is sometimes a reason why women prefer to pay privately for an abortion rather than seek an NHS referral from their general practitioner. Women and their doctors need to understand that contraception is not always easy to use and contraceptive 'accidents' are a fact of life — even for those who try to use a method carefully.

Table 1 Failure rates of commonly used contraceptives (1982 Oxford/FPA study data)[1]

Contraception method	Failure/100 women years
Combined pill	0.3
Diaphragm	1.9
Condom	3.6
Spermicide alone	11.9
Periodic abstinence (natural methods)	15.5

Effective use of contraception

The effective use of contraception depends on a combination of the following:

- consistency of compliance
- knowledge and skills
- circumstances in which sex takes place
- motivation.

Consistency of compliance

Most methods of contraception depend on their being used consistently according to instructions. Compliance is particularly an issue for users of oral contraceptives. A MORI poll, commissioned by the manufacturers of Norplant, found that 60% of 326 pill users had forgotten to taken their pill at least once during the preceding 12 months, while a further 7% were unable to say with certainty that they had always remembered.[8] Similar results have been obtained in other studies involving pill users, including in polls commissioned by manufacturers of oral contraceptives.

In an examination of the use of barrier methods, a recent study concluded that correct and consistent use relies on a complex interaction of the characteristics of the:

- methods themselves — extent of interference with sexual spontaneity and enjoyment, amount of partner cooperation required and ability to protect against sexually transmitted infections
- users — motivation to avoid unintended pregnancy, ability to plan, comfort with sexuality and previous contraceptive usage
- situational contexts — stage of sexual career, relationship characteristics and coercive elements such as physical or sexual abuse.[9]

Compliance is a difficult issue for reproductive healthcare workers to address. Research carried out by behavioural scientists, psychologists and sociologists suggests that compliance and non-compliance in all aspects of medical treatment — not just contraception — is a complex area of behaviour. Even when people are taking medicine that has an obvious beneficial effect, such as the relief of symptoms, compliance is often poor if the medicine is used over a long period of time. McGavock suggests that 20% of the population are 'highly compliant' and take medication precisely according to instructions, 40% comply reasonably well and 40% 'comply so badly that they achieve absolutely no benefit'.[10]

Users of oral contraceptives may be more motivated to comply than users of other long-term medication, as they have chosen to use this form of contraception instead of a long-acting or barrier method. However, some of the reasons for non-compliance identified by McGavock could be expected to apply:

- forgetfulness
- failure to understand the need to maintain use
- dislike of side-effects
- worries about long-term use.

A recent study of pill compliance among women aged 16–30 from Denmark, France, Italy, Portugal and the UK suggests that poor compliance was associated with a lack of established routine for pill-taking, failure to read and understand written materials that came with the contraceptives and occurrence of side-effects.[11] Women who were inconsistent pill takers, frequently missing one or more pills per cycle, were almost threefold as likely to experience an unintended pregnancy than women who took their pills consistently.

Table 2 Failure rates of commonly used contraceptives (1988 US National Survey of Family Growth data)[2]

Contraception method	Failure/100 women years
Combined pill	8
Diaphragm	16
Condom	15
Spermicide alone	25
Periodic abstinence (natural methods)	26

Some of these issues should be resolvable through better education, information and prescribing practice but, although suggesting that women who establish pill-taking 'habits' can reduce forgetfulness, it is unlikely that even the best doctor can completely eliminate non-compliance.

Knowledge and skills

Health professionals and contraceptive users often underestimate the level of knowledge and skills required to use contraception effectively. These are often, and wrongly, seen as issues solely for young people with little sexual experience.

A US study has shown that, although 80% of a sample of more than 3,000 people attending a genitourinary clinic said they were somewhat or very sure that they could put a condom on and take it off correctly, only 60% managed to demonstrate their perceived level of skill.[12] Anecdotal evidence suggests that problems with condom use are more likely to occur with 'reluctant users' — couples who would have preferred to use another method of contraception. This could be why events such as 'pill scares' can have a dramatic effect on the rate of unintended pregnancies, as couples who may have chosen to use the pill feel obliged to abandon a method of contraception that suited their sexuality and lifestyle and must reluctantly learn a new sexual etiquette.

Methods that can be dealt with in a methodical and routine fashion away from the distractions of sexual excitement are also associated with problems, even for well-informed women. For example, a woman may be aware that sickness and diarrhoea may interrupt the action of oral contraception, but it might still be difficult for her to judge whether or not her own illness was severe enough to make a difference. She may know that some antibiotics can undermine her contraceptive's effectiveness, but not which ones. A woman may know that she needs to use spermicide with her diaphragm, but may be unsure as to how much.

Circumstances in which sex takes place

Sex is still surrounded by stigma and taboos. The possibility of sex may be something that neither partner may wish to admit, especially if the relationship is in its early stages, or one or both partners feel uncomfortable about sex in general or their sexuality in particular. It is often suggested that people who are emotionally uncomfortable about sex are more likely to have unplanned pregnancies because they are less likely to:

- possess accurate information about conception and contraception
- acknowledge that they may have sex in the near future
- take steps to obtain contraception
- talk about sex with their partner
- use a chosen method of contraception consistently.

However, it should be accepted that even those who are completely comfortable with their sexuality, are well-informed about contraception and are able to communicate well with their partner may fail to use contraception effectively. Sex is not always prepared for and planned — nor do people always want it to be. The thought of spontaneous, passionate, impulsive, unpremeditated sex may be a nightmare for family planning doctors — but for many people it is the ideal dream! Sometimes sex happens and people take a chance; they may or may not become pregnant. It is prudish and judgemental to regard unprotected sex as necessarily inappropriate or dysfunctional behaviour.

Motivation

Effective use of contraception requires exceptional motivation. Since the chance of pregnancy with a single act of intercourse at mid-cycle is less than 30%, more than 70% of women will not become pregnant when contraception is not used. To expect consistent use of contraception to protect against unwanted pregnancy in the case of every act of intercourse during a woman's fertile life may be more demanding than most women can deliver.

Table 3 Reasons for not using adequate contraception[13]

Reason	Percentage
I didn't mind getting pregnant	20
I wanted to get pregnant	17
Contraceptive failure	12

Motivation to avoid pregnancy is a particularly important issue to address in respect of teenage pregnancy. A US study has concluded that 'the absence of negative attitudes towards having babies rather than negative attitudes towards contraception is the most commonly cited reason for non-use of contraceptives among childbearing adolescents'.[13] The most frequently cited reasons for not using adequate contraception in this survey of 200 adolescents are listed in Table 3.[13]

Such responses suggest that programmes aimed at reducing the number of unintended teenage pregnancies need to focus on issues other than sex education and access to contraceptive information and supplies. Instead, policy makers may need to consider why it is that young motherhood is seen as a positive option.

Conclusion

Long-acting methods that can be almost forgotten by the user once fitted are the most effective reversible contraceptives. Oral contraceptives taken as a matter of habit are less effective but are more likely to be used effectively than barrier methods which rely on either an anticipation of lust (diaphragms and caps) or an expression of lust (condoms). This has consequences for 'safer sex' messages.

Women who switch from hormonal to barrier methods of contraception may be placing themselves at a higher risk of unintended pregnancy and should be aware of appropriate strategies to deal with episodes of unprotected sex.

Post-coital contraception remains undervalued as a means of reducing the rate of unintended pregnancy. If it were conveniently available and widely advertised, it could provide a 'second chance' for women who think they have risked becoming pregnant. Currently, its potential is undermined by the fact that women are usually only able to obtain it by visiting a doctor within 72 hours of unprotected sex. The inconvenience of this may act as a significant disincentive to women. Evidence suggests that it would be safe and appropriate to provide emergency contraception through pharmacies without the need for a prescription.[14] If appropriate regulatory changes could not be made to allow this, it would make sense for doctors to prescribe emergency contraception to women in advance of their need to use it.[15]

Finally, policy makers need to accept that although the prevention of pregnancies is preferable to the termination of pregnancies, legal, easily available abortion is essential if couples are to regulate their fertility and plan their families. The number of unintended, unwanted pregnancies may be reduced by improvements in contraceptive techniques, and public knowledge of them, but it is unrealistic to imagine that 'family planning' can be achieved by contraception alone.

References

1. Vessey M, Lawless M, Yeats D. Efficacy of different contraceptive methods. *Lancet* 1982; **1**: 841–2.
2. Jones EF, Forrest JD. Contraceptive failure rates based on the 1988 National Survey of Family Growth. *Fam Plan Perspect* 1992; **24**: 12–9.
3. Fleissig A. Unintended pregnancy and the use of contraception: changes from 1984 to 1989. *BMJ* 1991; **302**: 147.
4. Bromham DR, Cartmill RSV. Are current sources of contraceptive advice adequate to meet changes in contraceptive practice? A study of patients requesting termination of pregnancy. *Br J Fam Plan* 1993; **19**: 179–83.
5. Lewis C, Wood C, Randall S. Unplanned pregnancy: is contraceptive failure predictable? *Br J Fam Plan* 1996; **22**(1): 16–9.

6. Murty J, Firth S. The use of contraception by women seeking termination of pregnancy. *Br J Fam Plan* 1996; **22**(1): 6–8.

7. Wheble AM, Street P, Wheble SM. Contraception: failure in practice. *Br J Fam Plan* 1987; **13**: 40–5.

8. MORI Consumer Survey. Survey of 1,257 women aged 16 to 49 throughout the UK, conducted in March and April 1993 on behalf of Roussel Laboratories Ltd.

9. Beckman LG, Harvey SM. Factors affecting the consistent use of barrier methods of contraception. *Obstet Gynaecol* 1996; **88**(3): 65–71.

10. McGavock H. Why don't patients comply? Improving patient compliance. *Pulse* 1998.

11. Rosenburg MJ, Waugh MS, Meehan TE. Use and misuse of oral contraceptives – risk indicators for poor pill taking and discontinuation. *Contraception* 1995; **51**: 283–8.

12. Langer LM, Zimmerman RS, Cabral RJ. Perceived versus actual condom skills among clients at sexually transmitted disease clinics. Public Health Reports 1994; **109**(5): 683–6.

13. Steven S, Simon C, Kelly L *et al*. Why pregnant adolescents say they did not use contraceptives prior to conception. *J Adolesc Health* 1996; **19**: 48–53.

14. Glasier A. Emergency contraception – time for deregulation? *Br J Obstet Gynaecol* 1993; **100**: 611–2.

15. Glasier A, Baird DT. The effects of self-administering emergency contraception. *N Engl J Med* 1998; **339**: 1–4.

Hormonal contraception

Anna Glasier, Family Planning and Well Woman Services, Edinburgh

Hormonal contraception has been available for nearly 40 years. Worldwide, hormonal contraception, and particularly the combined oral contraceptive pill, is used by more than 100 million women. In the UK, there cannot be many women who do not use hormonal contraception at some stage of their reproductive lives.

This paper will review important data, published during the past two years, of clinical relevance to the day-to-day management of women using hormonal contraception.

Combined oral contraceptive pill

The 'pill scare' of October 1995 arose from the impending publication of a number of studies,[1-3] which suggested that combined oral contraceptive pills (COCPs) containing a third-generation progestogen (desogestrel or gestodene) were associated with a higher risk of venous thromboembolism (VTE) than pills containing a second-generation progestogen, such as levonorgestrel. The relative risk of VTE compared with so-called second-generation pills varied from 1.5 to 3.1. Although the absolute risk of VTE is small and, even among women using third-generation pills, considerably less than the risk conferred by pregnancy, the UK Committee on Safety of Medicines (CSM) issued the advice that combined pills containing gestodene or desogestrel should be considered a 'second-choice' pill and should not be used at all by women with known risk factors for VTE, including obesity.

Much has been published since the appearance of the original studies. All the data were reviewed by a group of experts meeting at the World Health Organization in November 1997, and the report of this meeting is an extremely useful summary of the risks of cardiovascular disease among women using steroid hormone contraception.[4] The main conclusions of the group are described below.

Acute myocardial infarction

Acute myocardial infarction (MI) is uncommon in women of reproductive age. Its risk is not increased among pill users who do not smoke and do not have either hypertension or diabetes, regardless of age. Women who have hypertension and take the COCP have an increased relative risk of MI of at least threefold that of women who are normotensive and take the COCP. Smoking increases the risk of MI by 10-fold compared with non-smoking COCP users. There is insufficient evidence to reach any conclusion on whether or not the risk of MI is influenced by the type or dose of progestogen.

The implications of these findings are important to doctors and nurses advising women about the safety of the COCP. Women without risk factors can be reassured that no increased MI risk exists, regardless of their age.

Stroke

Ischaemic and haemorrhagic stroke are both uncommon among women of reproductive age.

The risk of ischaemic stroke is increased by about 1.5-fold in women who take the COCP, do not smoke and are not hypertensive. In contrast, the risk of haemorrhagic stroke in these women is not increased until they reach the age of 35, after which the increasing natural risk of haemorrhagic stroke is magnified by COCP use. Hypertension increases the risk of both ischaemic (by threefold) and haemorrhagic (10-fold) stroke when compared with never users.

Smoking increases the risk of ischaemic and haemorrhagic stroke (two to threefold) compared with pill users who do not smoke. There is insufficient evidence to determine whether the risk of either type of stroke is influenced by type or dose of progestogen.

Once again, the implications for healthy pill users are reassuring. Although the relative risk of ischaemic stroke is slightly increased, the absolute risk is very small. For women who are hypertensive or who smoke, the risk of MI and both types of stroke is significantly increased by the COCP. These women should be advised to use other methods of contraception and encouraged to stop smoking.

Venous thromboembolism

The risk of VTE is increased by three to sixfold among COCP users compared with non-users, but falls rapidly when COCP usage is stopped. The risk is not related to oestrogen dose in women using COCPs containing less than 50 μg ethinyl oestradiol. Pills containing deso-gestrel and gestodene probably carry a small risk of VTE beyond that of pills containing levonorgestrel. The absolute risk of VTE attributable to COCP use increases with age, obesity, recent surgery and some thrombophilias. The risk of VTE is unaffected by smoking or hyper-tension.

In April 1999, the CSM removed the restrictions placed in 1995 on the prescribing of third-generation oral contraceptive pills. The CSM has advised women be made aware of the existing data. Before the restrictions were lifted, some doctors switched women using third-generation pills to pills containing norgestimate. There are insufficient data to determine the effect of this pill on the risk of VTE but it is either similar to gestodene or desogestrel, or is an expensive alternative to levonorgestrel. There is no evidence to support widespread screening for inherited thrombophilias in women wishing to start using the COCP. Despite a number of publications on the effect of third-generation pills on the risk of MI, the statistical power of the studies is insufficient to demonstrate a convincing result.

Combined pill and breast cancer

A large meta-analysis published in 1996 demonstrates that the risk of diagnosed breast cancer is increased among women using the COCP (relative risk 1.24).[5] With time, after stopping the COCP, this increased risk declines but does not reach that of never-users until 10 years after stopping. Ever-users of the COCP who do develop breast cancer, however, have a decreased risk of metastases (relative risk 0.8).

These facts do not help to explain why there is an association between the COCP and breast cancer. The risk is neither dose-dependent nor dependent on the duration of use and the relationship, therefore, does not seem to be causal. It appears that either COCP use is associated with increased detection of breast cancer or, perhaps more likely, with late-stage promotion of malignant change.

New formulations

Recognizing concerns about the risks of long-term use of oestrogen, the pharmaceutical industry continues to seek the lowest dose of oral contraception that is both safe and effective. In an attempt to improve both efficacy and cycle control with a combined pill containing 20 μg ethinyloestradiol, Mircette has been launched in the US. Mercilon (20 μg ethinyloestradiol and 150 μg desogestrel) is followed by two days of placebo and then five days of 10 μg ethinyloestradiol before a new packet is started. There is evidence that this regimen is associated with less frequent resumption of follicular development during the pill free interval.[6] It seems likely that it would be associated with a higher incidence of amenor-rhoea which many women find worrying.

Progestogen-only pill

It has long been assumed that the progestogen-only pill (POP) has fewer long-term risks than the COCP because it does not contain oestrogen. Data have been scarce because the POP is not as commonly used. In 1998, however, the World Health Organization published a multinational study demonstrating no significant increase in the risk of acute MI, stroke or VTE among POP users or women using Depo-Provera.[7]

Depo-Provera

Two papers published in the early 1990s draw attention to the possible detrimental effect of long-term use of Depo-Provera on bone mineral density (BMD).[8,9] Since depot medroxyprogesterone acetate (DMPA) inhibits ovarian activity, a reduction in BMD, as a result of hypo-oestrogenism, is biologically plausible. The two studies showed that long-term use of DMPA resulted in BMD loss which partially recovered after stopping the method. A cross-sectional study from the UK of 185 women using Depo-Provera for more than five years, or amenorrhoeic after one year of use, showed only a minimal change in BMD which was unlikely to be of clinical significance.[10] Also in 1998, a study from New Zealand was unable to detect any significant difference in BMD when past-users were compared with controls.[11] Concerns remain, however, about the use of DMPA in adolescents who have yet to achieve their peak bone mass.

Contraceptive implants

Norplant has probably now found its place on the contraceptive menu in the UK. Although the pending litigation collapsed, Norplant manufacturers have decided to cease its marketing from autumn 1999 — it should be noted that this decision was not related to its safety or efficacy. In our clinic, continuation rates after four years of use of Norplant are over 65%.

The new single-rod desogestrel implant (Implanon) will be launched in Europe this year. Designed to last for three years, the dose of progestogen used inhibits ovulation in almost all users (in contrast to Norplant) and thus should be associated with a slightly higher incidence of amenorrhoea. The single rod and disposable inserter will make insertion and removal considerably easier.

Levonorgestrel-releasing intrauterine system

The levonorgestrel-releasing intrauterine system (Mirena) has been available in the UK for over two years. It is now licensed to last for five years and is a useful addition to the contraceptive formulary. In our hands significant numbers of women tend to exchange menorrhagia for frequent spotting but if they are properly counselled most find this more acceptable. Insertion of this rather large device can be facilitated by pretreatment with misopristol which has been shown to dilate the non-pregnant cervix.[12]

New delivery systems

Combined contraceptive patches and rings are currently in phase III trials throughout Europe and both look promising in terms of efficacy, bleeding patterns and acceptability.

Progestin-only gels and patches are at an earlier stage of development.

Conclusion

Hormonal contraceptives continue to be the most popular method of contraception in the UK. Recently published studies provide reassuring evidence for their long-term safety. Recent and future advances in delivery systems for contraceptive steroids give women greater contraceptive choice which should enhance acceptability and compliance.

References

1. World Health Organization Collaborative Study of Cardiovascular Disease and Steroid Hormone Contraception. Effect of different progestogens in low-oestrogen oral contraceptives on venous thromboembolic disease. *Lancet* 1995; **346**:1582–8.

2. Jick H, Jick SS, Gurewich V *et al*. Risk of idiopathic cardiovascular death and non-fatal venous thromboembolism in women using oral contraceptives with differing progestagen components. *Lancet* 1995; **346**: 1589–93.

3. Bloemenkamp KWM, Rosendaal FR, Helmerhorst FM *et al*. Enhancement by factor V Leiden mutation of risk of deep-vein thrombosis associated with oral contraceptives containing a third generation progestagen. *Lancet* 1995; **346**: 1593–6.

4. World Health Organization. *Cardiovascular disease and steroid hormone contraception*. World Health Organization Technical Report Series no 877. Geneva, WHO, 1998.

5. Collaborative Group on Hormonal Factors in Breast Cancer. Breast cancer and hormonal contraceptives: collaborative re-analysis of individual data on 53, 297 women with breast cancer and 100, 239 women without breast cancer from 54 epidemiological studies. *Lancet* 1996; **347**: 1717–27.

6. Killick SR, Fitzgerald C, Davis A. Ovarian activity in women taking an oral contraceptive containing 20 mg ethinyl estradiol and 150 mg desogestrel: Effects of low estrogen doses during the hormone-free interval. *Am J Obstet Gynaecol* 1998; **179**: S18–24.

7. World Health Organization Collaborative Study of Cardiovascular Disease and Steroid Hormone Contraception. Cardiovascular disease and use of oral and injectable progestogen-only contraceptives and combined injectable contraceptives. Results of an international, multicentre, case-control study. *Contraception* 1998; **57**: 315–24.

8. Cundy T, Evans M, Roberts H *et al*. Bone density in women receiving depot medroxyprogesterone acetate for contraception. *BMJ* 1991; **303**: 13–6.

9. Cundy T, Cornish J, Evans MC *et al*. Recovery of bone density in women receiving depot medroxyprogesterone acetate for contraception. *BMJ* 1994; **308**: 247–8.

10. Gbolade B, Ellis S, Murby B *et al*. Bone density in long-term users of depot medroxyprogesterone acetate. *Br J Obstet Gynaecol* 1998; **105**: 790–4.

11. Orr-Walker BJ, Evans M, Ames R *et al*. The effect of past use of the injectable contraceptive depot medroxyprogesterone acetate on bone mineral density in normal women. *Clin Endocrinol* 1998; **49**: 615–8.

12. Ngai SW, Chan YM, Liu KL, Ho PC. Oral misoprostol for cervical priming in non-pregnant women. *Hum Reprod* 1997; **12**: 2373–5.

Emergency contraception

Ali Kubba, Department of Obstetrics and Gynaecology, Guy's, King's and St Thomas' School of Medicine, London

Emergency contraception has been described as the best kept secret in family planning. Worldwide, there is poor awareness of this important emergency method and its provision remains extremely patchy and passive. This fact sits uncomfortably against a background of a clear need. The impulsive, liberating nature of sexual activity means that it can never be rationally controlled and planned on every occasion. It is, therefore, not surprising that in 1994 up to 49% of pregnancies in the US were unintended. The figure for teenagers was 79%.[1] All reversible contraceptives in current use are imperfect and many are user-dependent. Discontinuation is the extreme expression of unacceptability of particular methods to their users. A more prevalent trend is where users occasionally 'opt out' of the use of the method, putting themselves at risk of pregnancy. The more user-dependent the method, the more is this likely to happen. Users of methods such as coitus interruptus, condoms and fertility awareness would recognize any risk-taking events. Emergency contraception may be seen as complementing the user's chosen method, enhancing its efficacy.

In one survey, 70% of those requesting an abortion would have prevented an unplanned pregnancy if they had accessed emergency contraception.[2] Indeed, emergency contraception would have been used by 90% of a group of women requesting termination of pregnancy. Their access to this method was hindered by lack of awareness.[3]

Two methods

There are two broad categories: hormonal methods and copper intrauterine devices (IUDs). The use of vaginal douches or postcoital spermicides is unlikely to be effective as spermatozoa travel too quickly for such methods, accessing endocervical mucus within 90 seconds of ejaculation and are retrievable from tubal washings within five minutes of deposition in the vagina.

Hormonal

Of the hormonal methods, the combined oestrogen/progestogen method, popularized by Albert Yuzpe,[4,5] has been the dominant postcoital contraception technique used in the western world. Progestogen-only emergency contraceptives have been widely used in eastern Europe, China and some developing countries. Among the many progestogen-only regimens, the levonorgestrel one popularized by Ho and Kwan is emerging as the most effective.[6]

The antiprogesterone, mifepristone, proved a highly effective postcoital contraceptive in two World Health Organization-sponsored trials.[7,8] It was given as a single dose of 600 mg within 72 hours of unprotected intercourse. It exhibited a low risk of gastrointestinal side-effects but tended to delay the onset of subsequent menses due to a delay in ovulation. The longer treatment-menses period is seen as a disadvantage as couples may run further risks of contraceptive accidents or unprotected intercourse. Recurrent/regular use of mifepristone is likely to lead to menstrual chaos.

Combined hormonal emergency contraception (combined emergency pills)

Oestrogen/progestogen combined pills are administered in two doses. Each dose contains 100 μg ethinyloestradiol plus 1,000 μg norgestrel which is equivalent to 500 μg levonorgestrel. The first dose should be taken within 72 hours of intercourse, followed by the second dose 12 hours later. The method is effective throughout the 72-hour window but recent work by the World Health Organization shows higher efficacy with earlier treatment.[9]

The main side-effects of the combined method are gastrointestinal; nausea has been reported in up to 66% of users and vomiting in up to 24%. Other minor side-effects include mastalgia and headaches.

Emergency contraception may cause a change in the timing of the post-treatment menses. Menstruation occurs early in 15–20% of users, is late in 20% and is on time in over 50%; 98% of users would have had a period within three weeks of treatment.[4, 5]

The mechanism of action of hormonal emergency contraception, be it combined or progestogen-only (discussed below), is likely to be multifocal at ovarian, endometrial and tubal levels. The endometrium is 'de-synchronized' through an effect on endometrial enzymes and endometrial progesterone receptors, which are significantly down-regulated.[10] The endometrium is, therefore, rendered unreceptive to a fertilized ovum. These are the only consistently reported 'effects'. Many authorities in the field believe that transient disruption of ovarian activity is the most important action of the combined method. When given preovulation, hormonal methods tend to delay ovulation by approximately seven days and would prolong the cycle in question.[11] Given at, or after, ovulation the ovarian effect is variable but predominantly luteolytic.[12] Both oestrogens and progestogens affect tubal motility and this action may interfere with sperm and ovum transport and fertilization.

Progestogen-only emergency contraception

There is a long history of postcoital use of progestogens alone. This form of emergency contraception was originally introduced for repeated use following coitus, providing a simple, easy to teach method which promotes compliance in the less motivated. In such cases, coital frequency defines the exposure to hormones with a likely reduction in the total dose if coital frequency is restricted by protocol or the lifestyle of the user (eg the levonorgestrel product, Postinor, has a use limit of four times/cycle).

Several progestogen-only regimens have been used as emergency contraceptives. Efficacy was perceived to be inferior to the combined regimen until the publication of the Ho and Kwan comparative study confirming comparable efficacy to the Yuzpe method.[6] In 1998, a large, well conducted World Health Organization trial, comparing levonorgestrel-alone and the combined 'Yuzpe' regimens, revealed an efficacy of the levonorgestrel regimen higher than in earlier studies and surpassing the highest efficacy stated for the Yuzpe regimen.[9] Efficacy is likely to be higher with higher frequency of use.

Other advantages of progestogen-only emergency contraception are the absence of oestrogen, the lower risk of gastrointestinal side-effects and, possibly, being especially suitable for lactating women. There is a variable effect of progestogens on ovarian function. They can inhibit ovulation if used in frequent high doses.

Intrauterine devices

Postcoital use of copper-bearing IUDs started in the late 1960s. While hormonal methods are effective when used up to 72 hours after unprotected intercourse, emergency IUDs prevent pregnancies at least partly through inhibition of implantation of a fertilized ovum and remain highly effective when used up to five days from the earliest calculated date of ovulation.[13]

When efficacy is calculated per cycle of treatment, the emergency IUD has the lowest failure rate of all postcoital agents (under 1%). Only half a dozen failures have been reported in the literature comprising over 8,000 women-cycles.

The mechanism of action is hypothesized to be through the blastocidal action of copper and the prevention of implantation. Hormone-releasing intrauterine systems are not suitable for emergency contraception as copper, through its effect on endometrial enzymes, seems to be important for the spermicidal and antifertilization/implantation effect of the emergency IUD.[13] Studies seeking evidence of implantation in emergency IUD users have failed to detect β-human chorionic gonadotrophin. This refutes the notion that postcoital IUDs are abortifacient.

The emergency IUD is versatile in that it can be used up to five days from the earliest calculated date of ovulation (up to day 19 of a 28-day cycle, assuming that ovulation occurred on day 14).[13] This also means that an IUD can cover multiple exposures as long as they have all occurred within this time window. The use of the IUD up to seven days from unprotected intercourse was tested in a couple of studies but no conclusions can be drawn because of the small numbers involved.

The usual precautions that underpin IUD-use protocols apply to postcoital use. It is especially important to screen and/or administer prophylactic antibiotics in situations where there is risk of sexually transmitted infections, such as when unprotected intercourse has taken place with a new partner, was the result of a casual encounter or a sexual assault.

The classic contraindications to the use of the IUD, such as menorrhagia or a past history of ectopic pregnancy, do not apply to the use of the IUD postcoitally as the device is only required in the latter half of the cycle of treatment and, indeed, may be removed with the next menses. However, an advantage of the IUD is that it will serve as a contraceptive for the rest of the cycle of treatment and may be kept in situ for ongoing contraception if this is the woman's wish.

When used in young nulliparous women, consideration should be given to the use of local anaesthesia. Choice of device may be more important with a preference for devices with a small insertion diameter, such as the recently introduced Gynefix.

Relative efficacy

Failure of emergency contraception can be expressed in two ways. Crude failure rates are based on the percentage of treatment failures per cycle. A more accurate assessment of failure is to calculate the ratio of the pregnancies observed to those which would have been expected if a postcoital agent was not given.[14]

The IUD is the most effective emergency contraceptive with a failure rate of under 1%. The World Health Organization's randomized controlled trial comparing the Yuzpe regimen with the progestogen-only regimen confirmed the efficacy of the former, but showed it to be lower than in earlier studies. Although the World Health Organization trial had the advantage of large numbers (nearly 1,000 in each group) and fairly tight confidence intervals, its findings need confirmation. The overall failure rate of the Yuzpe regimen in this study was 3.2%, which is equivalent to a true efficacy rate of 57% (ie at least one in two pregnancies are prevented). In the same study, the efficacies of the Yuzpe and levonorgestrel regimens in a subset of 1,157 women who used the assigned regimens correctly were 76% and 89%, respectively. The fact that, in the whole group, the Yuzpe regimen was less effective makes one suspect that side-effects may have led some users to violate the protocol but not to report this to the investigators.

An important finding of the World Health Organization study, suspected by many earlier researchers, is the effect of the 'coitus-treatment' interval. Treatment early within the 72-hour window was more effective than treating late, the pregnancy rate being 2% in the first 24-hour and 4.7% in the past 24-hour window. The same study found the levonorgestrel-alone regimen to be highly effective when given up to 72 hours after unprotected intercourse. The overall failure rate is 1.1% with a significant trend of higher efficacy the earlier the treatment is given (0.4% in the first 24 hours rising to 2.7% in the past 24 hours of the 72-hour window). The incidence of gastrointestinal side-effects was also less with levonorgestrel-alone. Ethnic origin did not affect efficacy.

Recurrent use

The total dose of the Yuzpe regimen is equivalent to seven low-dose combined oral contraceptive pills. The levonorgestrel-alone method has 50% more progestogen but the total dose is still relatively low. Even if used repeatedly, the total dose would be small compared to regular pill taking. There is no evidence to suggest that women resort to emergency contraception in place of ongoing regular family planning. Those women who may experience recurrent episodes of unprotected intercourse or contraceptive failure may be best served by emergency contraception to avoid an unplanned pregnancy and should not be denied the treatment.

Antiemetics

In case of vomiting within two hours of ingestion of the tablets, a repeat dose with an antiemetic is recommended, or the use of an IUD should be considered. The optimal antiemetic is domperidone because of its safety profile and the lack of extrapyramidal side-effects or sedation. Domperidone acts on the chemoreceptor trigger zone, which is the area that triggers nausea and vomiting in hormonal method users.

Antiemetics do reduce the risk of nausea and vomiting. Routine concomitant use of antiemetics has been associated, in one study, with a lower failure rate.[15]

Drug interaction

Broad-spectrum antibiotics are unlikely to have an impact on bioavailability of the contra-ceptive steroids so no alteration of the dosage is required. Drugs that induce hepatic enzymes may be expected to reduce bioavailability and, thereby, efficacy. It is recommended in those taking such drugs that the dose of the Yuzpe regimen is increased by 50% (ie three tablets used within 72 hours and repeated 12 hours later, instead of two tablets).

The future

Mifepristone remains a promising product, whose true potential is untested. It has the attraction of a single dose being non-oestrogenic with high efficacy and low gastrointestinal side-effects.

The true potential of emergency contraception in reducing unplanned pregnancies and abortions is still unrealized as a result of poor awareness and motivation from some health professionals and the public in many parts of the world. The fact that emergency contra-ception remains a prescription medication is a barrier against wider use, although one also has to address the manufacturers' anxiety about uncontrolled use and the potential for liti-gation. A compromise solution may be the provision of emergency hormonal contraception through pharmacists following a local, regional or national protocol and liaising with local healthcare providers.

Self-administration/'take home' emergency contraception is likely to support responsible use of effective contraception. The largest study in this area confirms that making emergency contraception available for self-administration does not reduce the use of other mainstream methods of contraception.[16] In the study, the relative risk of unintended pregnancies was 0.7 in the self-administering group compared to controls. Although this result was not statistically significant, it points to a potential advantage of making emergency contraception more easily available.

The concept of a 'once a month' hormonal contraceptive is unlikely to be practical because of the need to time the treatment accurately for mid-cycle/ovulation suppressing methods or the ethical considerations of the use of a once a month method late in the cycle.

Acknowledgements

This paper is broadly based on Kubba A, Guillebaud J. Emergency contraception. In: Kubba A, Sanfilippo J, Hampton N, eds. *Contraception and office gynecology*. London: WB Saunders, 1999.

References

1. Henshaw SK. Unplanned pregnancy in the United States. *Famil Plann Perspect* 1998; **30**: 24–9, 46.
2. Duncan G, Harper C, Ashwell E *et al.* Termination of pregnancy: lessons for prevention. *Br J Famil Plann* 1990; **15**: 112–7.
3. Bromham DR, Cartmill RS. Knowledge and use of emergency contraception among patients requesting termination of pregnancy. *BMJ* 1993; **306**: 556–7.

4. Yuzpe AA, Lance WJ. Ethinylestradiol and dl-norgestrel as a post-coital contraceptive. *Fertil Steril* 1977; **28**: 932–6.

5. Yuzpe AA, Percival Smith R, Rademaker AW. A multi-centre clinical investigation employing ethinylestradiol combined with dl-norgestrel as a post-coital contraceptive agent. *Fertil Steril* 1982; **37**: 508–13.

6. Ho PC, Kwan MSW. A prospective, randomised comparison of levonorgestrel with the Yuzpe regimen in post-coital contraception. *Hum Reprod* 1993; **8**: 389–92.

7. Glasier A, Thong KJ, Dewar M, Baird DT. Mifepristone (RU 486) compared with high dose estrogen and progestogen for emergency post-coital contraception. *N Engl J Med* 1992; **327**: 1041–4.

8. Webb AMC, Russell J, Elstein M. Comparison of the Yuzpe regimen, Danazol and mifepristone (RU 486) in oral post-coital contraception. *Br J Med* 1992; **305**: 927–31.

9. Task Force on Postovulatory Method of Fertility Regulation. Randomised, controlled trial of levonorgestrel versus the Yuzpe regimen of combined oral contraceptives for emergency contraception. *Lancet* 1998; **352**: 428–33.

10. Kubba AA, White JO, Guillebaud J *et al*. The biochemistry of human endometrium after two regimens of post-coital contraception: A dl-norgestrel/ethinylestradiol combination or danazol. *Fertil Steril* 1986; **45**: 512–6.

11. Ling WY, Wrixon W, Acorn T *et al*. Mode of action of dl-norgestrel and ethinyl estradiol combination in post-coital contraception. III. Effect of preovulatory administration following luteinizing hormone surge on ovarian steroidogenesis. *Fertil Steril* 1983; **40**: 631–6.

12. Ling WY, Wrixon W, Zayid I *et al*. Mode of action of dl-norgestrel and ethinyl-estradiol combination in post-coital contraception. II. Effect of postovulatory administration on ovarian function and endometrium. *Fertil Steril* 1983; **39**: 292–7.

13. Kubba A, Wilkinson C. *Recommendation for clinical practice: emergency contraception*. London: Faculty of Family Planning and Reproductive Health Care, 1998.

14. Kubba A. The efficacy of emergency hormonal contraception. In: Paintin D, ed. *The provision of emergency hormonal contraception*. London: RCOG Press, 1995.

15. Baghshaw SN, Edwards D, Tucker AK. Ethinyl oestradiol and dl-norgestrel is an effective emergency post-coital contraceptive: A report of its use in 1,200 patients in a family planning clinic. *Aust NZ J Obstet Gynecol* 1988; **28**:137–40.

16. Glasier A, Baird D. The effects of self-administering emergency contraception. *N Engl J Med* 1998; **339**:1–4.

Risk communication

Michael Campbell, University of Sheffield, Sheffield

All medical procedures carry a risk; a risk-free intervention does not exist. It is important for doctors and other health professionals to understand how risk is measured, since they have to interpret information from government agencies and drug companies. It is also important for them to be able to communicate the magnitude of the risk of an intervention so that patients can meaningfully appraise their treatment options. Thus, there are two aspects of risk communication:

- communicating with other professionals
- communicating with patients.

Communicating with professionals

Agencies such as the Committee on Safety of Medicines (CSM) inform the medical profession about the risks of certain drugs.

Four concepts need to be understood: risk, relative risk (RR), absolute risk reduction (ARR), and the number needed to treat (NNT).

In a cohort of people, some are exposed to a hazard while others are not. The *risk* of an event, such as death, is expressed as the number of events occurring in a group divided by the length of time the cohort has been followed-up. The *relative risk* is the ratio of the risk in the exposed group to the risk in the unexposed group. For example, the risk of a venous thrombotic event in those taking a third-generation oral contraceptive (low dose) is 30 per 100,000 women years, and for second-generation oral contraceptives it is 15 per 100,000 women years (Table 1). Thus, the relative risk is 30/15 = 2. The *absolute risk reduction* is the difference between the two risks and is given by 30–15 = 15 per 100,000 women years. The *number needed to treat* is the inverse of the ARR, ie 6,700 women years. The interpretation of this is that 6,700 women would each have to take the third-generation oral contraceptive pill for one year, for one additional woman to suffer a deep venous thrombosis (DVT). In an ideal world, confidence intervals would be attached to these estimates to indicate how precisely they have been estimated, but uncertainty about an uncertainty estimate is hard to grasp. In general, one needs to know both the absolute risk and the relative risk in order to convey information about risk adequately.

The consequences of the CSM warning about third-generation combined oral contraceptives in 1995 was an increase in the number of legal abortions, from 39,000 in the quarter before the warning to 45,000 in the succeeding quarter. As can be seen from Table 1, pregnancy carries a much higher risk of a thrombotic event (or DVT) than being on the low-dose pill.

Other questions asked by general practitioners interpreting these data may include:

- To what extent is the increased risk a consequence of simply swapping formulations, and that perhaps a swap from third- to second-generation contraceptives may also carry a risk?

Table 1 Risks associated with the use of oral contraceptives[1]

	Venous thrombotic episodes/ 100,000 women/year
Oral contraceptive not used	5
Use of pill (second-generation)	15
Use of low-dose pill (third-generation)	30
Pregnancy	60

- How long does the risk last? Is it possible that it persists for only a short period of time and that those who do not react quickly are unlikely to react at all?
- To what extent are the results due to selective prescribing such that women perceived to be at high risk were selectively prescribed the third-generation oral contraceptives?

Recent research has shown that over a 25-year follow-up, the relative risk of death for ever-users versus never-users of oral contraceptives was 1.0 (95% CI 0.9 to 1.1).[2] For women who were current or recent users (< 10 years), there was an increased risk of cervical cancer and cerebrovascular disease, but a reduced risk of ovarian cancer. Women who had stopped taking the pill for more than 10 years had no significant excesses or deficits for any specific cause of death.

Many professionals still do not understand the way risk is communicated. Fahey *et al* presented the same piece of research evidence about the effectiveness of mammography screening to executive and non-executive members of 13 health authorities in four different ways: relative risk reduction, absolute risk reduction, proportion of event-free patients and the number of patients needed to be treated.[3] The willingness to fund a new programme was significantly influenced by the way the data were presented. The relative risk (which gives larger absolute numbers) produced the highest score in terms of willingness to fund. Only three (of 140) recognized that the summary measures all related to the same piece of evidence!

Communicating with patients

Research has shown that patients (and indeed most of the population) have a very poor understanding of risk.[4] Most daily activities, such as commuting to work, smoking or drinking alcohol, carry risks. Different daily activities carry very different risks which are often not appreciated by the public. Research has shown that it is usually not worth communicating risks numerically. Risk applies to groups: individual patients will either get the disease or not, and their belief in the likelihood of this event is only partially tempered by the true risks. Otherwise why do people smoke and buy lottery tickets?

Many authors suggest that the best way to communicate risk is to relate it to the risks associated with daily activities, and to grade it with descriptions such as 'moderate' or 'low'.

Table 2   The Calman Chart.[1] Risk of an individual dying (D) in one year or developing an adverse response (A)

Term used	Risk range	Example	Risk estimate
High	> 1:100	(A) Transmission to susceptible household contacts of measles and chickenpox	1:1–1:2
		(A) Transmission of HIV from mother to child (Europe)	1:6
Moderate	1:100–1:1 000	(D) Smoking 10 cigarettes per day	1:200
		(D) All natural causes, age 40	1:850
Low	1:1 000– 1:10,000	(D) All types of violence	1:3,300
		(D) Influenza	1:5,000
		(D) Road accident	1:8,000
Very low	1:10,000– 1:100,000	(D) Leukaemia	1:12,000
		(D) Playing soccer	1:25,000
		(D) Accident at work	1:43,000
Minimal	1:100,000– 1:1,000,000	(D) Accident on railway	1:500,000
Negligible	< 1:1,000,000	(D) Hit by lightning	1:10,000,000
		(D) Release of radiation by nuclear power station	1:10,000,000

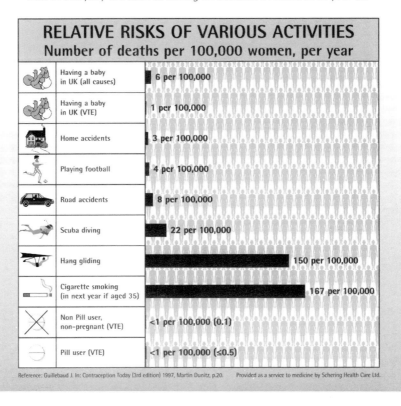

PATIENT INFORMATION
THE PILL AND VTE

Venous thromboembolism (or VTE, for short) is a condition where blood clots develop in the veins (usually in the legs)

○

Women taking the Pill have a slightly greater risk of VTE than women not on the Pill, but the risk is much lower than the risk in pregnancy

○

The risk of dying as a result of VTE is still much lower compared with other risks in everyday life such as having an accident at home or in your car

RELATIVE RISKS OF VARIOUS ACTIVITIES
Number of deaths per 100,000 women, per year

	Having a baby in UK (all causes)	6 per 100,000
	Having a baby in UK (VTE)	1 per 100,000
	Home accidents	3 per 100,000
	Playing football	4 per 100,000
	Road accidents	8 per 100,000
	Scuba diving	22 per 100,000
	Hang gliding	150 per 100,000
	Cigarette smoking (in next year if aged 35)	167 per 100,000
	Non Pill user, non-pregnant (VTE)	<1 per 100,000 (0.1)
	Pill user (VTE)	<1 per 100,000 (≤0.5)

Reference: Guillebaud J. In: Contraception Today (3rd edition) 1997, Martin Dunitz, p.20.   Provided as a service to medicine by Schering Health Care Ltd.

Figure 1: The Schering chart providing information on the pill.
Reproduced with permission[5]

Examples of this are the Calman Chart,[1] the Paling Perspective Scale[4] and the Schering Chart,[5] the latter being designed particularly for oral contraceptives. The Calman Chart (Table 2) grades risk into six bands from 'high' (> 1:100) to 'negligible' (< 1:1,000,000). The Paling Perspective Scale has 13 bands and scores on the logarithm of risk that are adjusted so 'Home Base' — the baseline to which all other risks are referred — is a risk of 1 in 100,000. The Schering Chart (Figure 1) includes a bar chart showing magnitude of risk, as well as numbers. This replaces the 1991 version.

Edwards *et al* studied the Calman Chart, the Paling Perspective Scale and the 1991 version of the Schering Chart as a means of communicating risk in primary care; the professional opinion was that they are not ideal for communicating risk to the general public, although the Schering Chart was appreciated for its visual method of conveying risk.[6] Problems include differentiating between voluntary and involuntary risk, and between fatal and minor outcomes. For example, people felt with the Schering Chart that it would be better to compare alternative methods of contraception, since there was an element of choice, whereas there was no alternative to crossing the road. People are much more likely to accept risks that are taken voluntarily. Also missing from the equation is the benefit to the individual from taking the risk; smokers and hang-gliders regard the benefit of their activities as outweighing the risks involved. Drugs often carry a risk of side-effects but these are acceptable for the sake of a cure. None of the above-stated methods consider the number of people likely to be affected, which forms the basis of decisions made by Public Health professionals. Statisticians have attempted to do this, looking at deaths resulting from large-scale catastrophes, but the results are not very sensible.[7]

Risks are also subject to fashion. The risk of death due to meningitis has not changed recently, but it is now customary for newspapers to report deaths of students from meningitis over the winter. The fear of child molesters has instituted major social changes in the way children are taken to school and in their social activities, despite the lack of evidence that it is any more dangerous for children to be out of doors than it was 50 years ago. Other fashions have come and gone, without noticeable change in the underlying risk, such as listeria and necrotizing fasciitis. Currently there is concern about new variant CJD, which carries a risk of 1 in 2,000,000, and because of the Bristol scandal, the risk of surgery. Patients will start demanding comparative risk figures for different surgeons in the same way as they require school performance figures, although it will be difficult to communicate this risk to the public in a meaningful way.

When risks are unavoidable but controllable, then a consensus has to be developed as to what is acceptable. Thus there is a consensus on speed limits and levels of toxins in drinking water.

Conclusion

No medical procedure is completely safe and patients should be informed in a clear and non-alarmist way about the level of risk. There is need for an ongoing debate about medical risks, and work to elaborate these for many medical procedures. A method of communicating these risks meaningfully to the public is also required.

References

1. Calman KC. Cancer: science and society and the communication of risk. *BMJ* 1996; **313**: 799–802.
2. Beral V, Hermon C, Kay C *et al*. Mortality associated with oral contraceptive use: 25-year follow-up of cohort of 46,000 women from Royal College of General Practitioners' oral contraceptive study. *BMJ* 1999; **318**: 96–100.
3. Fahey T, Griffiths S, Peters TJ. Evidence based purchasing: understanding results of clinical trials and systematic reviews. *BMJ* 1995; **311**: 1056–60.
4. Paling J, Paling S. *Up to your armpits in alligators*. Florida: John Paling and Co Ltd, 1996.
5. Guillebaud J. *Contraception today*. 3rd ed. London: Martin Dunitz, 1997: 20.
6. Edwards A, Matthews E, Pill R, Bloor M. Communication about risk: the responses of primary care professionals to standardizing the 'language of risk' and communication tools. *Famil Pract* 1998; **15**: 301–7.
7. Duckworth F. The quantification of risk. *RSS News* 1998; **Oct**: 10–12.

Patient communication

Toni Belfield, Family Planning Association, London

To communicate is defined as 'to impart (knowledge) or exchange (thoughts, feelings, or ideas) by speech, writing, gestures' (Collins).

Increasing knowledge and confidence depend on providing accurate, complete, accessible, consistent and memorable information. One of the forces driving the concept of evidence-based patient choice is the wish to provide people with information. The value of patient information is enormous and research demonstrates consistently that providing useful information enables people to make choices. Patient choices and behaviour do not simply depend on the provision of information, but how the information is presented and how people are involved in the decision-making process.

Contraception, sexual and reproductive health, more than any other branches of medicine, are areas where the relationship between the professional and the public is important. Recognizing the dynamics between professionals and patients and providing useful, accessible information contributes to this partnership. Through this, informed choices and decisions can be made which recognize the complexity of people's lives and the multiplicity of psychosocial factors influencing decision and choice.

This paper will focus on professional (doctor/nurse)–patient communication and how this relates to contraception and sexual health, and determine ways of improving the presentation of contraceptive information.

Information revolution

For years, medicines were prescribed and dispensed with little or no information; it was assumed that people would not be interested or have the intelligence or understanding to benefit from receiving information about their treatment or drugs. Today, there is a revolution in patient information. Involving people in the management of their health by enabling or empowering them through information provision, and the parallel growth of patient and advocacy groups, have resulted in people having access to information from a variety or sources. Some sources are accurate, providing up-to-date and impartial information; many are not, providing inaccurate, misleading and sometimes sensationalist misinformation. The growth and wider availability of the Internet provides for more information; however, much of this is inaccurate and misleading.[1] The value of patient information is enormous and research demonstrates that providing information has beneficial effects as well as enabling people to make choices.[2,3]

Information needs

The last half of this century has seen enormous changes in the availability and provision of contraceptive methods and services. Research shows that people are knowledgeable about contraception. However, considerable research throughout the world demonstrates consistently that both men and women still lack knowledge about:

- from where to obtain contraception (particularly emergency contraception)
- choice of contraceptive methods
- how contraceptive methods work
- risks and benefits of methods
- what to do if a method fails or if a method's efficacy is compromised.

As a result, unintended pregnancies and requests for abortion remain high.

Contraceptive methods are not perfect and they do fail even among the most careful of users. All methods can have adverse effects which are often well publicized and can discourage use. Oral contraception, while by far the most commonly used reversible contraceptive method, is the most talked about, worried about and misunderstood drug. It is also one of the most researched drugs, but public confidence about its use is low. Research suggests women do not administer it correctly, consistently forget to take it, and are not aware of its true risks and benefits. This lack of knowledge can be positively identified with compliance.[4–6]

Women's and men's contraceptive needs, expectations and choices are influenced by many factors, including: knowledge, information, lifestyle, age, religion, ethnicity and perceptions (their own and others'), anxieties and embarrassment.[7–9] Provider preference and service delivery contribute to limiting or improving acceptability and choice.[2,10] The ability to control fertility has been shown to be directly related to the amount of information an individual has, how they feel about their sexuality and sexual identity, as well as feelings of personal self-worth and determination.[7]

Promoting knowledge and confidence

To increase knowledge and confidence on contraception depends on the ability of the professional to identify and counter misinformation, and to promote the benefits of use through accurate, complete and consistent information. Patient choices are not solely dependent on the provision of information, but also on their involvement in decision making and how the information is understood. For people to participate fully in decision making they need to be authorized to ask questions, to make demands, to make informed decisions *and* be able to consent.

The provision of good contraception and sexual health services requires training and support, knowledge, skill and sensitivity. How we communicate greatly influences the adequacy of the contraceptive consultation and its outcomes. For example:

- are we friendly/welcoming?
- do we ask questions?
- how do we ask questions?
- do we use appropriate language?
- do we listen?
- are we aware of our non-verbal communication?
- do we take enough care when providing a contraceptive method or during physical examinations?

These factors affect patient satisfaction, confidence and compliance.

Many professionals make assumptions, often underestimating a person's degree of motivation, ability or needs, and 'censor' or limit information; many pressure a woman to use certain methods. As a result, women express feelings of anger, frustration and powerlessness because they feel they are not being heard, spoken to on equal terms and given time or permission to voice fears or anxieties. These findings are supported by the daily enquiries to the UK Family Planning Association's national Helpline; the helpline responds to more than 100,000 enquiries a year on all aspects of contraception, sexual and reproductive health.

Research shows that women and men want *more* information, not less.[2,7] This is in direct contrast to the opinion of a number of professionals who feel that the public cannot deal with 'too much' information. Clearly, people have a right to be informed of certain information, such as advantages, disadvantages and the uncertain areas about risk and benefit and information they *need* to know in order to use their chosen method safely and effectively.

Informed choice

Professionals need to be aware of the extent of their role in determining a choice rather than influencing it. Hatcher *et al* address informed choice and consent as having three bases:[11]

- *pragmatically*: a person who understands their contraceptive method is more likely to use it safely and effectively
- *ethically:* every person has the right to know about methods and procedures that can affect their health
- *legally:* information must be given so people can make an informed decision.

Strategies to improve service delivery

Recognizing the complexities in contraceptive choice, a number of strategies can be introduced to address and improve the way in which contraceptive information is discussed and delivered.[12]

Contraceptive service provision

Strategies to improve the service of providing information include:

- Provide accessible and flexible clinical services that address the diversity of sexual and reproductive healthcare needs within the community.
- Provide a full range of contraceptive methods or accessible referral to other services that do.
- Ensure all staff (medical and non-medical) are appropriately trained, updated, supported and resourced — use a combination of different skills.
- Provide information about services so people *know* about them.
- Ensure confidentiality in visits, communications and record keeping. This is important for all age groups but especially for teenagers, where aspects of confidentiality outweigh any anxieties about the consequences of unprotected sex.[13–15] Staff should sign a confidentiality clause.
- Practise an ethos of equality regarding age, gender, race, sexual orientation and disability.
- Ensure an established rapport and mutual respect with clients is maintained.
- Ensure consulting rooms are pleasant and do not have barriers (ie desks) between the professional and client.
- Provide sufficient *time* for contraceptive consultations, especially for the first visit.
- Provide, where appropriate, a choice of male or female doctors, advocacy workers and interpreters.
- Provide effective services that are designed, developed and delivered on the basis of local needs assessment, which include the views of users, past users and non-users of services.
- Provide efficient and good quality audited services.
- Know of other sexual and reproductive health services, for referral.

Contraceptive information and counselling

Various strategies to improve the way in which information and advice are provided include:

- Recognize that contraception and sex are inextricably linked (as one cannot be discussed without the other) and that, for many, this may be embarrassing and a cause of anxiety, inhibiting them from seeking information and advice.
- Always provide accurate, complete, objective and consistent information.
- Use suitable, appropriate language that enables and informs (talk about intrauterine devices (IUDs) not coils, progestogen-only pills not minipills, fertility awareness methods not rhythm, emergency contraception not morning after pills).
- Be aware and note non-verbal cues such as body language, tone of voice, speed of talking.
- Always discuss risks, benefits and uncertainties. All information and advice should be explicitly supported by the best available evidence.
- Be a catalyst and facilitator, not an 'educator' who tends to tell the client what needs to be done. Determine information needs and concerns by asking questions.

- Recognize that people are not always comfortable and need 'permission' to ask questions. Listen to the client and respond.
- Spend more time on compliance-related issues at the initial consultation.
- Provide useful, accessible, verbal information and written information to support advice on methods, recognizing that a client's questions and answers are based on:
  - effectiveness, ie will the method work? There is no perfect method and providing information about contraceptive efficacy is complex. Research by the Family Planning Association illustrates the need to present this information in both percentages and numbers with definitions.[16] This must also recognize the need to discuss the difference between 'user' and 'method' failure rates.
  - suitability, ie will it cause harm?
  - risks and benefits, known and unknown.
  - how to use a method, ie when to start using a method, when it becomes effective, when to stop its use (eg for planned pregnancy), how long it can be used for.
  - what to do if a method fails, is not used consistently, is concomitantly used with other drugs or illness.
  - how the method works, ie do its primary or secondary actions prevent ovulation or work before or after ovulation? This has important considerations for those who believe that life begins at fertilization, rather than the general medical and legal opinion defining life as beginning at implantation.
- Increase motivation — be prepared to offer solutions to practical difficulties the client experiences in using methods correctly and consistently (such as provision of written information or telephone support).
- Be aware of clients not attending follow-up or not collecting repeat prescriptions.
- Recognize that a compliant attitude does not necessarily reflect compliant behaviour.
- Recognize that non-compliance may result from feelings or loss of status and/or control.
- Pay attention to discussed side-effects (whether or not real or perceived).
- Discuss the transient nature of side-effects that relate to hormonal methods when starting a method (ie unpredictable bleeding).

Conclusion

Obtaining harmonized, objective, information on reproduction and fertility is not only a necessity but is also a right. Such knowledge: provides an understanding of how health, emotions and behaviours relate to fertility; enables an unravelling of the myths, misconceptions and misinformation that exist; and can minimize the embarrassment and anxieties surrounding this often taboo subject. Good medical practice relates to mutual respect between the professional and client, good information sharing and high quality, continuity of care. Knowledge and choice on contraception give empowerment and confidence which, in turn, enables improved reproductive decisions and choices to be made.

References

1. Wyatt JC. Measuring quality and impact of worldwide web. *BMJ* 1997; **314**: 79–81.
2. Walsh J, Lythgoe H, Peckham S. *Contraceptive choices — supporting effective use of methods*. London: Family Planning Association, 1996.
3. Coulter A. Evidence based patient information — is important, so there needs to be a national strategy to ensure it'. *BMJ* 1998; **317**: 225–6.
4. ESC. International Working Group on Enhancing Patient Compliance and Oral Contraceptive Efficacy — consensus statement. *ESC Newsletter* 1992; **2**: 1–4.
5. Rosenberg M, Waugh MS, Long S. Unintended pregnancies and use, misuse and discontinuation of oral contraceptives. *J Reprod Med* 1995; **40**: 355–60.
6. Rosenberg M, Waugh MS. Causes and consequences of oral contraceptive noncompliance. *Am J Obstet Gynaecol* 1999; **180**(2): 276–9.

7. Belfield T. Consumer perceptions of family planning. *Br J Famil Plann* 1988; **13**(4): 46–53.

8. Oddens BJ. *Determinants of contraceptive use: national population-based studies in various Western European countries*. International Health Foundation. Eburon Publishers, 1996.

9. Ravindran Sundari TK, Berer M, Cottingham J. Beyond acceptability: Users' perspectives on contraception. Reproductive Health Matters for WHO. *Reproductive Health Matters*, 1997.

10. Belfield T. Problems of compliance in contraception. *Br J Sex Med* 1992; **19**(3): 76–8.

11. Hatcher RA, Trussell J, Stewart F *et al*. *Contraceptive technology*. New York: Irvington Publishers Inc, 1994.

12. Belfield T. The contraceptive decision — information and counselling. In: Kubba A, Hampton N, Sanfilipo J, eds. Contraception and office gynaecology: Choices in reproductive health care. London: WB Saunders, 1999.

13. Hadley A. Private and confidential. *Women's Health* 1997; **2**(1): 20–2.

14. Brook Advisory Centres. *Someone with a smile would be your best bet – what young people want from sex advice services*. London: Brook Advisory Centres, 1998.

15. Kishen M. Adolescent contraception. *Diplomate* 1997; **4**(3): 207–13.

16. Godwin K. Consumers' understanding of contraceptive efficacy. *Br J Famil Plann* 1997; **23**(2): 45–6.

Non-hormonal methods

Walli Bounds, Margaret Pyke Centre and University College London, London

Non-hormonal methods, comprising intrauterine devices (IUDs), male and female barrier devices, spermicides, natural family planning and lactational amenorrhoea, are invaluable contraceptive options, both for short- and long-term use. Their relative freedom from health risks is particularly appealing to the health-conscious user. This paper will focus on the current thinking of and technological advances in these methods.

Intrauterine devices

IUDs, widely accepted in the 1970s and 1980s, are now regrettably much underused in the UK, largely due to adverse media publicity. They provide highly effective, convenient, reversible, long-term contraception at relatively low cost. Indeed, modern copper IUDs, such as the T Cu-380A, TCu220C and MLCu-375, are at least as effective as injectables and female sterilization.[1] Thus, they are particularly suitable for women interested in sterilization but are at increased risk of regret, eg aged under 30 years.

Mirena

The more recently introduced progestogen-releasing intrauterine system, Mirena, is especially suitable for women with pre-existing menorrhagia and/or dysmenorrhoea. It may eventually become available for other gynaecological indications,[2] although in the UK it is currently only licensed for contraception. Mirena needs to be replaced after five years, irrespective of the woman's age at the time of insertion; copper IUDs can be left in situ until the menopause if fitted after age 40.[3]

Gynefix

Gynefix, a frameless IUD consisting of six tiny copper beads attached to a nylon thread, is the latest addition to the range of IUDs available in the UK. Good efficacy, less pain/bleeding and low expulsion rates are its potential benefits, but more randomized comparative trials are needed to substantiate these claims. Careful patient selection, ideally combined with Chlamydia screening, skilful insertion and supportive monitoring thereafter, are the key to success with any IUD and with Mirena.

Apart from long-term contraceptives, copper IUDs are the most effective method of emergency contraception. If used for this indication, the insertion needs to be undertaken within five days of unprotected intercourse. Where the earliest episode of unprotected intercourse was more than five days previously, an IUD can still be fitted, in good faith, up to five days after the calculated earliest day of ovulation.[4]

Condoms

Condoms are highly effective contraceptives if used consistently and correctly. They also play an important role in preventing the transmission of sexually transmitted infections (STIs), mainly human immunodeficiency virus (HIV).[5] This, combined with their ease of availability and freedom from needing medical intervention, make condoms particularly suitable for couples at the start of a sexual relationship. In addition, they are ideal short-term contraceptives, eg while considering or waiting to start a more permanent method.

Improvements in manufacturing techniques and quality control, such as the introduction of the European Standard BS EN 600, have resulted in high-quality products. Other recent advances include greater choices in condom design (shapes, textures, colours, sizes) in order to meet consumer preferences and the introduction of a polyurethane condom (Avanti), suitable for those with latex rubber allergy. Avanti is thinner and wider than latex rubber condoms. A randomized comparative trial showed it to be the preferred choice among nearly one-half of the 360 participants,[6] but its relatively high cost limits more widespread use. Other variants of polyurethane condoms are undergoing trials but are not yet commercially available in the UK.

Of female condoms under development, to date only one variant (Femidom) is generally available. Made from polyurethane, loose-fitting in design, and extending over the vulva, it is particularly useful for women at high risk of STIs and for those with latex rubber allergy. Clinical trials suggest Femidom's effectiveness in preventing pregnancy is in the range of that reported for male condoms.[7,8] Familiarization with the method and sustained and correct use are essential for success.

Diaphragms and caps

Diaphragms and cervical caps are small rubber devices designed to occlude the cervix. They are held in place by a metal spring incorporated in the rim (diaphragms) or by suction (cervical caps). All need to be fitted by trained personnel and used in combination with a spermicide. Claims that a diaphragm pre-soaked in honey and used without a spermicide (known as a 'Honeycap') is as effective as a diaphragm used in combination with a spermicide, are not supported by scientific evidence.[9] Careful selection of the most appropriate type and size of device and thorough education on its correct use are essential. Apart from affording effective contraception, if used consistently and correctly, female occlusive devices give some protection against pelvic infection and cervical cell abnormalities, which may explain their popularity among health conscious women.

New variants, designed for over-the-counter use with no or only minimal formal teaching, include the Lea's Shield, Oves Cap and Femcap. All three are made of silicone rubber, incorporate a removal loop, and need to be used in conjunction with a spermicide. They differ from each other in physical configuration, size and thickness of the silicone material. While the Lea's Shield is more akin to a diaphragm, the remaining two are variants of cervical caps. To date, these devices have undergone only limited clinical trials and therefore reliable efficacy data are not yet available. Lea's Shield and Oves Cap are already marketed in selected European countries and have undergone the now mandatory European Union 'CE-Marking' assessment. However, since the 'CE-Marking' is primarily an assessment of product safety (ie risk to health), it should not be interpreted as a guarantee of clinical effectiveness.

Spermicides

Spermicides in current use are mostly surfactants, nonoxynol-9 being the most widely used worldwide. Although only moderately effective when used alone, they have a role in pregnancy prevention, especially as adjuncts. Spermicides are presented in a variety of base materials (cream, jelly, pessary and pressurised foam), although lack of good comparative trials make assessment of their relative efficacy and acceptability difficult. Patient preferences seem to be the deciding factor in choosing a particular type.

Spermicides also have bactericidal and virucidal properties, demonstrated in numerous in vitro and in vivo studies and thus have a role in STI prevention.[10] While in vitro studies have shown nonoxynol-9 can inactivate HIV, clinical trials have failed to confirm a protective effect. Research into other spermicides/virucides, including chlorhexidine, cholic acid and dextrin sulphate, is underway.

Natural family planning

Natural family planning (NFP), comprising the calendar, temperature and mucus method, or a combination known as the symptothermal method, is a useful form of fertility regulation and is highly effective, provided unprotected intercourse is restricted to the postovulatory phase of the cycle. High motivation and meticulous adherence to the rules are essential for success. Ideally, those choosing this method should receive formal teaching by a qualified NFP instructor.

A recently introduced electronic device, Persona, which measures hormonal changes in urine, is 94% effective, but potential users need to understand its limitations. Failure to comprehend that '94% effective' still represents one pregnancy in 17 women, appears to have been the main reason for the recent controversy surrounding this product. Persona is contraindicated in women whose cycle length falls outside the range 23–35 days, who are breastfeeding, using hormonal treatments, have liver or kidney disease, menopausal symptoms or polycystic ovarian syndrome and who are on long-term tetracycline.

Lactational amenorrhoea method

The lactational amenorrhoea method (LAM) is a widely practised form of contraception worldwide, although it is relatively little used in the UK. Providing the woman is fully breast-feeding, amenorrhoeic and within six months following delivery, the pregnancy rate is only 2%.[11] As soon as any one of these conditions changes, alternative methods of contraception should be started.

Conclusion

All non-hormonal contraceptives play a crucial role in the prevention of unwanted pregnancies. Methods that additionally protect against STIs are of particular relevance to the young, sexually vulnerable sections of society. In view of their protective effect, their use should be more widely encouraged, as adjuncts to hormonal methods too.

References

1. Treiman K, Liskin L, Kois A et al. IUDs — an update. Population Reports 1995; **Series B** (6, 22): 1–33.
2. Sturridge F, Guillebaud J. Gynaecological aspects of the levonorgestrel-releasing intrauterine system. Br J Obstet Gynaecol 1997; **104**: 285–9.
3. Tacchi D. Long-term use of copper intrauterine devices. Lancet 1990; **336**: 182.
4. Kubba A, Wilkinson C. Emergency contraception update. Br J Famil Plann 1998; **23**: 135–7.
5. Cates W. How much do condoms protect against sexually transmitted diseases? IPPF Med Bull 1997; **31**: 2.
6. Frezieres RG, Walsh TL, Nelson AL et al. Breakage and acceptability of a polyurethane condom: a randomized, controlled study. Famil Plann Persp 1998; **30**: 73–8.
7. Bounds W, Guillebaud J, Newman GB. Female condom (Femidom). A clinical study of its use-effectiveness and patient acceptability. Br J Famil Plann 1992; **18**: 36–41.
8. Farr G, Gabelnick H, Sturgen K. et al. Contraceptive efficacy and acceptability of the female condom. Am J Public Health 1994; **84**: 1960–4.
9. Bounds W, Guillebaud J, Dominik R et al. The diaphragm with and without spermicide. A randomized, comparative efficacy trial. J Reprod Med 1995; **40**: 764–74.
10. Feldblum PJ, Fortney JA. Condoms, spermicides, and the transmission of the human immunodeficiency virus: A review of the literature. Am J Public Health 1988; **78**: 52–4.
11. Anonymous. Consensus statement. Breastfeeding as a family planning method. Lancet 1988; **2**: 1204–5.

Looking to the future

John Guillebaud, Margaret Pyke Centre, London

The negative publicity surrounding contraceptives since the 1970s has meant that contraceptive research and development has been seen as unprofitable. As predicted by Djerassi,[1] very few entirely new birth-control methods have emerged in recent years (Figure 1). The global population rises each year by around 80 million, hence more than 6,000 million, many utterly destitute, human beings will be living on this planet at the start of the next millennium. Human needs will never be met without stabilizing human numbers on a finite planet.

It is estimated that up to 64% of pregnancies worldwide are either timed incorrectly or totally unwanted. Therefore, a large proportion of the 580,000 maternal deaths occurring annually represent deaths, not only from unsafe abortions, but also full-term deliveries, which resulted from pregnancies the women never wanted.

This paper will focus on the requirements for ideal reversible contraceptive methods and possible contraceptive advances to be seen in the new millenium.[2]

Combined oral contraceptives

The pill will remain popular in the 21st century, regardless of the uncertainty triggered on October 18th 1995 by the Committee on Safety of Medicines (CSM) in the UK.[3] This was based on studies suggesting a doubling of the risk of venous thromboembolism with desogestrel (DSG)- or gestodene (GSD)-containing pills as compared with those containing levonorgestrel (LNG) or norethisterone (NET) and its pro-drugs. The extra annual risk was estimated as around 10 per 100,000, equating to a tiny excess mortality risk of around two per million, from venous thromboembolism. The differential risk has not been confirmed in more recent studies, but even if real, it is very small in comparison with those that are accepted in life generally.

Regardless of loss of confidence through 'pill scares', its supremacy in the contraceptive field is being increasingly challenged. A useful criterion for new methods is that the 'default state' should be contraception (rather than conception, as when the pill-user defaults!).

Mifepristone and other progesterone antagonists

Aside from research, products of this type are used solely for medical termination of pregnancy. However, mifepristone is close to 100% effective for postcoital contraception when used according to the same criteria as the existing combined oestrogen–progestogen approach, with far fewer women reporting side-effects. The only problem seems to be delay in the next menses and re-establishment of cycling, particularly among women treated before ovulation. Use of

Figure 1:
Possible reasons for the recent decline in development of new birth-control methods.
Reproduced with permission from Denis Lincoln

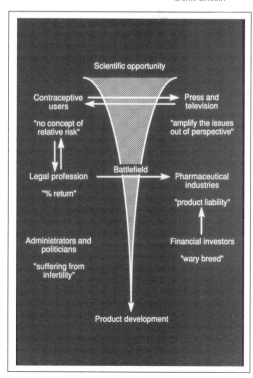

65

much lower doses helps to overcome this problem, and the effectiveness of the method may be extended to five days after coital exposure.

Studies are in progress in Edinburgh and elsewhere which may lead to methods of regular birth control. This could be by regular 'contragestion' which would interfere with implantation during the final days of the cycle and would, therefore, be rejected by some as abortifacient. However, mifepristone and other progesterone antagonists prove to be effective when small oral doses are used early in the cycle in such a way that they interfere with ovulation on a regular basis. The problems with bringing progesterone antagonists to the market, even for uncontroversial prefertilization applications, are not medical but legal and ethical.

Vaginal caps

There are two new, interesting vaginal caps (Lea's Shield and Femcap). These are more simple to use than the diaphragm and do not need to be clinically fitted, although both must be used with spermicides (Figure 2). Their efficacy is thought to be similar to that of a well-fitting diaphragm, and they are entering the market in some countries, although more efficacy data are awaited.

Condoms and spermicides

Female condoms

Figure 2: Two vaginal caps: (a) Femcap and (b) Lea's Shield

Femidom is currently on the market; this is known as Reality in the US. The 'bikini condom' failed dismally on aesthetic grounds, but the 'panty condom' — with a replaceable, lubricated, vaginal pouch secured to underwear — seems promising, and empowers the woman whose partner should but will not use a condom of the male variety.

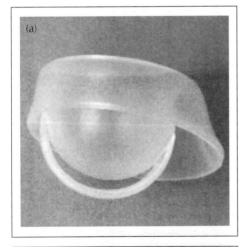

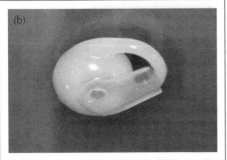

Viricides/spermicides

This approach has been ludicrously underfunded despite its huge potential benefit. The testing of many candidate compounds is under way, in the hope of identifying a substance which, in a suitable delivery system, will reduce if not eliminate virus transmission. It is relevant to consider user-friendly microbicides in the context of contraception, even if a successful product could not provide adequately effective contraceptive. This is chiefly because their use would enable potentially HIV-exposed couples to employ one of the more effective 'medical' methods of contraception, which would otherwise not be an option. Currently, male condoms are often used inexpertly for both contraception and HIV protection, leading to many unwanted conceptions.

Loose-fit internally lubricated male condoms

There is renewed interest in male condoms, partly through the observation that many men prefer the 'freedom' of coital movement within the female condom. Using both latex and polyurethane materials, various agencies are actively researching lubricated loose-fit male condoms in which the shaft and glans penis are allowed free movement. Ez-On is the first marketed product which is available in the Netherlands.

New hormone delivery systems for women

Injectables

Depot medroxyprogesterone acetate (DMPA) given as a dose of 150 mg every 12 weeks and norethisterone enanthate (NET-EN) 200 mg every two months are used worldwide. More recently, monthly combined injectables have been devised through the World Health Organization, working mainly in South America, and proving to be very popular. They lead to a bleeding episode approximately monthly and are highly effective.

The most promising product is Cyclofem (25 mg DMPA with 5 mg oestradiol cypionate). This can be delivered efficiently — a special self-injector helps to overcome the problem of the need for frequent clinic visits for the monthly injections. Advantages include the more regular bleeding pattern, lack of hypo-oestrogenic symptoms and potential risks, and the fact that patients who develop symptoms do not have to wait long for reversal to be achieved.

Subdermal progestogen implants

Norplant is likely to be supplanted in the UK by Implanon, a single ethylene vinyl acetate rod releasing 3-keto-desogestrel over three years;[4] similar single but biodegradable capsules are also expected to appear on the market. Implanon is easier to insert and remove than Norplant — it had an average removal time of 2.6 minutes. No failures have been reported in 2,300 insertions. As with all progestogen-only methods, its main remaining problem is the occurrence of irregular bleeding.

Vaginal rings

One version of a vaginal ring was close to being marketed in 1993, releasing levonorgestrel over a period of three months. In a study at the Margaret Pyke Centre, however, some erythematous vaginal patches were detected which, on histology, showed evidence of inflammation. It is not certain whether or not this was due solely to mechanical pressure, or a chemical or allergic reaction to either the levonorgestrel or the polymer.

The vaginal ring concept remains viable. The combined 3-keto-desogestrel and ethinyloestradiol ring, which is softer and more flexible than the levonorgestrel ring, appears most promising. Rings may also be potential vectors for microbicides.

Transdermal patches

Transdermal patches are currently marketed primarily for administering hormones for oestrogen replacement therapy. In the very near future, they will be used as an alternative to the pill.

Luteinizing hormone releasing hormone analogues and antagonists

Luteinizing hormone releasing hormone (LHRH) analogues and antagonists show potential for use both to ablate the menstrual cycle in women and to block spermatogenesis in men. In both sexes, there would be a need for add-back gonadal steroid treatment: oestradiol for women and testosterone for men. This would prevent the unacceptable side-effect of loss of libido (and hot flushes in women). In women it would also be necessary to protect the endometrium from over-stimulation and this could be done using the levonorgestrel-releasing intrauterine system (LNG-IUS), discussed later.

Other peptide-based approaches

There is potential to produce long-acting follicle-stimulating hormone (FSH)-receptor or human chorionic gonadotrophin (hCG)-receptor blockers to prevent follicular development or to block implantation, respectively. The same technology might also be used to block the action of peptides important in the complex process of sperm–oocyte fusion.

Systemic contraception approaches for men

Research on testosterone esters is currently under progress by the World Health Organization. These can either be used alone or in smaller doses in combination with progestogens. All can be given as long-acting injections or potentially by other routes such as subcutaneous implants. There is a risk that the testosterone-based methods might create an increased risk of arterial disease, prostatic hypertrophy or aggression, but careful titration of the doses is now minimizing such hazards.

There would be an advantage for compliance if any marketed product were not, in fact, a 'male pill': an injection or implant could be given or at least supervised by his more likely reliable partner!

Immune approaches in both sexes

The most advanced immune approach in Phase II trials is the method based on active immunity to hCG using the appropriate antigen plus adjuvants. However, this method has already been under development for 25 years without a reliable product emerging. Another approach being considered is immunity to the zona pellucida or to various sperm antigens. In the latter case, simulation of natural conditions in which a man is entirely healthy but his sperm fail to fertilize is intended. However, the approach appears likely to be more successful in women than by raising autoantibodies to the man's sperm.

With all the potential immune methods, the problem of individual variation is acute in that some individuals are poor responders so that conception results despite oft-repeated booster doses and others are hypersensitive with the risk of immuno-sterilization. The avoidance of the risk of (auto)-immune disorders is also a high priority.

Fertility awareness-based methods

In developed countries, these are likely to be more widely used through the development of better technology, both to predict and detect ovulation. A small, hand-held, electronic computer and urine-testing device called Persona has already been marketed (Figure 3). This predicts ovulation by placing a dipstick in the woman's urine; the first significant rise of oestrone-3-glucuronide is measured and a red light informs her that she is entering her fertile period. The end of this period (with return to a green light on the device) is detected from the luteinizing hormone surge followed by computer calculations of the time necessary for any ovulated egg to become non-fertilizable. In ongoing use, the system adapts to the individual woman by referring to her stored data for the previous six cycles.

Figure 3: Persona — the personal contraceptive system. Reproduced with permission from Unipath Ltd

From the main European trial, the current best estimate for the first-year failure rate among consistent users is 6/100 woman-years (Keith May of Unipath, personal communication). This makes it inappropriate for women who need greater efficacy, unless they are prepared to use barriers or abstain during the first 'green' phase (preovulatory phase, always less effective due to the capriciousness of sperm survival) , as well as the red one. It is also likely to prove prohibitively expensive for most Third World countries.

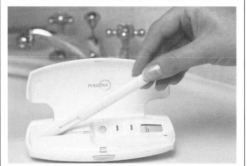

Intrauterine contraception

Copper intrauterine devices

Wildemeersch et al[5] have produced a banded copper delivery system (Gynefix) based on a single polypropylene thread bearing a knot, which is pushed by a special inserting stilette 1 cm into the fundal myometrium. Studies show that when the devices are properly inserted, this approach retains the excellent efficacy of the Copper T 380 and its derivatives, yet minimizes the risk of both expulsion and uterine pain. It also shows potential (with the knots enhanced in various ways) for immediate postabortal and postplacental insertion.

It is hoped that this technology might in due course be applied to silastic cylinders or threads releasing progestogenic hormones as, in the form already marketed (Mirena), intrauterine progestogen conveys many other advantages. I predict that this uterine implant technology will be a crucial ingredient of the contraceptive 'mix' of the 21st century.

Levonorgestrel-releasing intrauterine system (LNG-IUS, Mirena)

This releases 20 μg/24 hours of levonorgestrel (LNG) from its polydimethylsiloxane reservoir through a rate-limiting membrane. Its main contraceptive effects are local by endometrial suppression and changes to the cervical mucus and utero-tubal fluid which impair sperm migration. The blood levels of LNG are around one-quarter of the peak levels in users of the progestogen-only pill, so ovarian function is altered less. Most women continue to ovulate and, in the remainder, sufficient oestrogen for health is produced from the ovary even if they become amenorrhoeic, as many do: this is primarily a local end-organ effect and should be seen as a benefit. Postmenopausal oestradiol levels have not been detected even in those who have no uterine bleeding.

Clinical advantages and indications

I maintain that for most parous women this represents the future and it is already here although not so recognized by many providers. Combining most of the best features of hormonal and intrauterine contraception without most of the problems of either, it fundamentally rewrites the textbooks about IUDs. Advantages include:

- unsurpassed efficacy — less than 0.2 per 100 woman-years in the first year
- return of fertility is rapid and appears to be complete
- the user can expect a dramatic reduction in amount and, after the first few months (discussed below), in duration of blood loss. Dysmenorrhoea is also generally improved.

The LNG-IUS is certainly the contraceptive method of choice for most women with heavy menses or who are prone to iron-deficiency anaemia — a particularly relevant bonus to the Third World. It also shows promise for a number of gynaecological indications:

- a first-line treatment for frank menorrhagia
- as part of the management of severe premenstrual symptoms (PMS) with high-dose (100–200 μg) oestradiol skin patches
- possibly, to prevent fibroid growth, uterine pain from adenomyosis and endometrial hyperplasia
- in the perimenopausal woman, it provides progestogenic protection of the uterus during oestrogen replacement therapy by any chosen route.[6] Studies at the Margaret Pyke Centre and elsewhere confirm that this is a fully contraceptive regimen with most women achieving amenorrhoea whether the IUS is inserted before or after final ovarian failure and progestogenic (PMS-type) side-effects are very rare.

Main adverse effects

Like any IUD it can be expelled and there is the usual small risk of perforation, although this is minimized by its 'withdrawal' technique of insertion. The infection risk may be reduced but not entirely eliminated by its marked progestogenic effect on genital tract fluid. A more important problem is the high incidence in the first post-insertion months of uterine bleeding which, although small in quantity, may be very frequent or continuous and can cause considerable inconvenience. There is also a small incidence of steroidal side-effects, such as acne and breast tenderness. These tend to improve with time and forewarning helps.

Table 1 Main features of the 'ideal' contraceptive

• 100% reversible	• 100% protective against sexually transmitted infections
• 100% effective (with the 'default state' = contraception)	• Possessing other non-contraceptive benefits
• 100% convenient (discreet and non-coitally related)	• Non-medical, maintenance-free (needing no ongoing
• 100% free of adverse side-effects (neither risk nor nuisance)	medical intervention)

Conclusion

LNG-IUS fulfils many of the criteria for an 'ideal' contraceptive (Table 1), particularly once the thread-borne variant is available. There are few adverse side-effects and, in general, they are in the category of 'nuisance' rather than hazardous.

It is to be hoped that new contraceptives fulfilling even more completely the ideal criteria of Table 1 will be developed for widespread use in the 21st century. In particular, methods requiring no special skill to be applied/distributed, without nuisance side-effects and protective against sexually transmitted infections are needed. In the mean time, the LNG-IUS sets a high standard and, hopefully, a cheap price can soon be set for it in order to harness both its contraceptive and health benefits for the maximum possible number of women worldwide.

References

1. Djerassi C. *The politics of contraception*. WW Norton: New York, 1979.

2. Guillebaud J. Contraception for the 21st century. In: Johansson EDB, ed. *The levonorgestrel intrauterine system –The new contraceptive option for parous women*. Parthenon: Carnforth, 1998: 11–32.

3. Committee on Safety of Medicines. *Combined oral contraceptives and thromboembolism* (letter). CSM: London, October 18 1995.

4. Archer D, Kovacs L, Landgren BM. Implanon®, a new single rod contraceptive implant. *Contraception* 1998; **58**(6): 755–1155.

5. Wildemeersch D, Batar I, Webb A *et al*. Gynefix®. The frameless intrauterine contraceptive implant — an update. *Br J Fam Plann* 1999; **24**: 149–59.

6. Sutionen SP, Allonen M, Lahteenmaki P. Sustained-release oestradiol implants and a levonorgestrel-releasing intrauterine device in hormone replacement therapy. *Am J Obstet Gynecol* 1995; **172**: 562–7.

Index